Soccer

Nutrition

A Step-by-step Guide on How to Outsmart Your Opponents

(How to Quickly Transform Your Life and Game by Eating Like a Pro)

Robert Murphy

Published By **Cathy Nedrow**

Robert Murphy

All Rights Reserved

Soccer Nutrition: A Step-by-step Guide on How to Outsmart Your Opponents (How to Quickly Transform Your Life and Game by Eating Like a Pro)

ISBN   978-1-7774070-9-4

Published By **Cathy Nedrow**

ISBN   978-1-7774070-9-4

Legal & Disclaimer

Table Of Contents

Chapter 1: Carbohydrates

The gasoline furnished with the beneficial resource of carbohydrates is the most inexperienced for the manufacturing of electricity. Carbohydrates are stored as glycogen in muscular tissues and within the liver.

Most carbohydrates produce 'sluggish release' power. This is because of the truth your body does no longer eat them proper away.

In order to experience in shape and prepared to perform on the sector, it's far crucial that soccer gamers devour a respectable amount of top carbs previous to a hobby or exercising session.

When you are physically active, your muscle organizations gets maximum of the energy they need from stored glycogen. It is consequently important that your frame has suitable tiers of glycogen for the muscular tissues to apply after they maximum want it.

With inadequate portions of glycogen, your frame will soon start to tire, and your mental consciousness and coordination may additionally even go through because of this.

As a football participant, approximately 60% of your weight loss program wants to return from carbohydrates. Your healthy dietweight-reduction plan ought to embody small, however frequently-eaten, carb-wealthy food.

However, you want to don't forget at the identical time as making plans your diet that not all carbohydrates are properly. There are numerous forms of carbohydrates available within the immoderate road shops and you want to understand what's what.

The charge at which your frame breaks those carbs down and transforms them into glycogen differs considerably from one to the opposite. This is why you want to recognize your carbs. Fortunately, this is not a tough workout.

The breakdown-price of carbohydrates may be measured with the aid of using the glycemic index (or GI). Foods which characteristic immoderate on the glycemic index are broken down right away via manner of the body, while food lower on the size are broken down an awful lot slower.

Eating the incorrect form of carbohydrates at the wrong time of day might also have an effect to your overall performance on the sector. You need to carefully plan your carbohydrate consumption to make sure you bought and preserve top power stages.

For example, if you are gambling a activity within the overdue-afternoon, you have to really try to consume a big, unmarried-supporting of 'sluggish' carbohydrates 4 or five hours earlier than kick-off.

On the opposite hand, in case your game is scheduled for the morning, then you surely have to stock up your energy reserves with the useful resource of consuming a small amount of higher GI carbohydrates.

Just undergo in thoughts that having an suitable sufficient quantity of saved glycogen is essential in your ordinary overall performance within the route of a game.

Playing soccer includes hundreds of strolling spherical and distinct immoderate-strength actions, all of which could quick expend the body's glycogen levels.

Players who are properly stocked-up with glycogen ought to have a extraordinary advantage over any of their warring parties who aren't. Having enough glycogen way you'll be capable of run quicker, deal with more difficult, and undergo longer.

So that allows you to preserve your glycogen at the right degree you want to devour the right varieties of carbohydrates at the proper times, and additionally ensure you live hydrated via ingesting masses of fluids at normal periods. This is your recipe for success.

So what form of carbohydrates need to you be consuming, and at the same time as precisely?

Well, one famous desire amongst soccer gamers proper right here in my neighborhood Sweden, and a non-public preferred of mine, is pasta (carbohydrate) and meat sauce (protein/carb) taken four-5 hours earlier than a exercise.

This form of meal may be supplemented with bread, potatoes, and rice, followed by a serving of fruit (bananas are an exceptional, carb-rich preference).

These styles of carbohydrate characteristic approximately halfway at the glycemic index, that is why they will be nice consumed a few hours earlier than a undertaking.

If your endeavor starts offevolved earlier inside the day, then you need to eat some better GI carbs. I want to have muesli, milk, and raisins in this situation, as those food offer the fast energy improve I want for an early kickoff.

You will want to calculate the right blend of sluggish and speedy carbs to your weight loss plan. Don't worry, that is nowhere close to as fiddly, or as time ingesting, as it would sound.

In truth, once you get familiar with it all you will be knocking your everyday food up without giving a 2nd perception to the way. In the beginning despite the fact that, you could want to seek advice from a GI table, clearly till you grow to be familiar with which meals come beneath what class.

Carbohydrates are virtually important for retaining a right football weight-reduction plan. Without the right amount, or kinds, your body may be starved of the strength it desires, and that means you might not be capable of characteristic as you would like to.

Having brilliant technical capacity and nicely-evolved talents is important for all and sundry who wants to compete seriously in soccer.

But even in case you very very own outstanding potential, you can but not be able to take advantage of your abilties to their complete ability if your body and muscle tissue are not furnished with the proper type of gasoline.

So, if you recall that playing soccer is certainly approximately ability, then anticipate once more. Proper vitamins is a must-have, no longer a preference, or at the least not for extreme players.

1.1.1 Monosaccharides

Monosaccharides (from the Greek phrases monos: single, sacchar: sugar) are the most easy devices of carbohydrates.

They are the most effective shape of sugar and are colorless, water-soluble, crystalline solids. The list beneath includes a few examples of diverse kinds of monosaccharide:

Glucose (dextrose)

Fructose (laevulose)

Lactose

Xylose

Ribose

Your frame absorbs monosaccharides thru the cell wall that lines your small gut. From right right here, they're transported into the bloodstream from in which they get stored as electricity.

When monosaccharides stay within the body for too lengthy without being used for power, they're then transformed into fats and stored inside the fats tissue.

Fructose is an instance of this form of monosaccharide. The frame treats fructose in a different manner to exceptional carbohydrates.

Carbohydrates commonly bypass thru the liver, in which the body makes a selection whether or not or no longer to use them as electricity without delay or save them as glycogen for later use.

Yet research have validated that fructose bypasses the liver altogether and is instead right away metabolized with the aid of the body. Any quantity that is not required right now's then stored as glycogen.

Monosaccharides provide your frame with an exquisite, balanced form of strength. However, as with every meals, they want to be fed on most effective moderately.

1.1.2 Disaccharides

Disaccharides (which means ' sugars') are determined in nature as lactose, sucrose, and maltose. They are carbohydrates that function excessive-up at the glycemic index. This way they are suddenly broken down and for this reason purpose a pointy upward thrust in blood glucose ranges.

Sucrose, this is normal through the usage of glucose and fructose, is what's commonly used as table sugar.

Lactose is a key factor of milk (you may have heard of lactose-intolerance or milk hypersensitivity) and is formed with the beneficial useful resource of glucose and galactose.

Unlike lactose and glucose, maltose isn't a herbal substance, so it wishes to be made from one-of-a-type factors of carbohydrate.

1.1.Three Polysaccharides

Polysaccharides are complex carbohydrates. Complex carbohydrates are made from sugar molecules and may be placed in elements which include, beans, complete grains, peas, and wonderful vegetables. Because in their period, Polysaccharides are with out troubles converted into glucose strength (blood sugar) with the resource of the frame.

1.2 Protein

Protein is crucial for boom and tissue restore. It additionally enables to keep a robust immune tool. It is important for making essential enzymes and hormones. Protein is placed in its maximum concentrations in beef, nuts, fish, and milk.

Approximately 15% of your each day calorie consumption need to be long-mounted by means of protein. This will assist your frame to get better quicker after video video games and stay resilient in competition to injuries.

You might also were ordered with the useful resource of way of your educate subsequently to 'placed a few muscle on those bones' at the way to increase a more potent average usual performance on the world.

The simplest manner to do this is with the resource of way of ingesting enough protein. Protein is crucial for any attempts you're making to reinforce up.

It is the vital component trouble (on the side of workout) desired thru your muscle agencies to growth and become stronger.

Soccer players want to consume around 0.6 to 0.Eight grams of protein constant with pound of body weight, in step with day, as a manner to repair muscle mass, help muscle increase, and hold muscle energy.

Protein also can be utilized as a pre-match power booster, even though it received't provide you with same degree of strength reserves as carbohydrates.

While there are various manufacturers of protein merchandise, only a few of them use the crucial factors/procedures to ensure the producing of a tremendous protein that the frame dreams.

Indeed, some of the promotional spiel can, on some labels, of numerous merchandise, be quite misleading. To positioned it more bluntly, some companies offer merchandise that are not what they claim to be, so this without a doubt is a case of client watch out!

If you do plan to complement your protein consumption with dietary supplements, then you definately actually need to be cautious and research the marketplace properly in advance than looking for into some thing.

Make outstanding you most effective use a immoderate first-class product due to the fact it is able to be much less complicated to your body to take in and hire the components effectively.

A low wonderful protein product, as an alternative, have to pass right through your system with out consisting of any, or very little, gain in any respect, because of this making it now not anything greater than high priced urine.

There also are one-of-a-type kinds of protein merchandise. So which of those are notable appropriate for you and your goals? Well, that relies upon for your precise necessities. Below are a number of the more not unusual varieties of protein that you could want to check out.

1.2.2 Whey Protein

This is the most famous protein complement available within the marketplace these days. Whey protein generally is to be had in powder shape and is easy to dissolve in water. This makes it easy to put together, consume, and digest inside the body.

Whey protein ranks excessive in organic charge (BV), that could be a dimension this is used to decide how well your frame makes use of the nitrogen it strategies from the protein.

Without going too technical, actually understand that nitrogen is a essential nutrient this is used for muscle boom. Some research even declare that protein includes numerous additives which could absolutely enhance the frame's immune response.

1.2.Three Soy Protein

One reason why soy protein isn't always famous among football gamers is as it comes from a plant deliver. This method it does now not comprise all the vital amino acids which can be required for muscle increase.

Also, some of the number one soy merchandise available on the market were crude soy powders. These powders have been complete of sodium and carbohydrates.

However, this all-vegetable source of protein has prolonged lengthy long gone through some huge changes as it first hit the excessive streets.

Nowadays, soy protein includes complete protein, and moreover has one of the maximum inexperienced levels of digestibility of all protein sources.

Soy beans moreover incorporate very little fat and almost no cholesterol. If you are lactose illiberal, you ought to at the least bear in mind soy protein as it is honestly freed from lactose.

Some studies have even ranked soy protein better then red meat, milk, and eggs; despite the fact that in the wider scientific community, the jury stays out on that one.

1.2.Four Egg Protein

Eggs, seemed as an great deliver of protein, have featured cautiously in fitness and protein-intensive diets for the motive that early Nineteen Sixties.

Dense quantities of protein are found within the eggs whites, and because of this they'll be a excellent opportunity to meat.

Egg protein is likewise especially-digestible, with about ninety seven% of it being absorbed as amino acids, that might then be utilized by the frame to synthesize new protein.

1.Three Fat

Fat is frequently related to being fats or obese. This has led the substance to address bad connotations. It is pretty usually assumed that every one fats is awful for you, but it's not, as many professional football game enthusiasts, and one-of-a-kind athletes, will let you know.

Fat is a supply of important fatty acids which include omega-3. They are known as "essential" because the human body can not cause them to on its very own.

Around 25% of your healthy dietweight-reduction plan have to encompass fats. Fat is needed for boom and to and absorb vitamins and minerals.

However, not all fat are same, and not all fat are top to your health each, so some kinds need to be prevented. This is some thing that you truly do need to be aware of.

Other forms of fats, however, are appropriate for you. In fact, some kinds of fat are important for preserving a healthful weight-reduction plan.

Yet it can regularly be overwhelming whilst searching for to decipher which styles of fats are appropriate for you and people which are not.

Furthermore, some fat that are stated to be wholesome are recognizable with the aid of names like "Extra Virgin Olive Oil," for instance, but even a number of those may not be all that they seem.

This is because of the truth some producers, no matter the truth that now not all manufacturers, have other, dangerous fat brought to them, a few problem which is not continuously obvious or perhaps protected in the data.

To assist guide you on the numerous fat available I will describe the wonderful kinds with out the usage of too much technical jargon.

OK, there are essentially 3 high-quality sorts of fat, especially saturated fat, unsaturated fat, and trans fat.

Saturated fats are those which may be strong at room temperature. Foods excessive in saturated fats come especially from animals, even though lesser quantities can be located in some flora.

Unsaturated fat comes with some fitness advantages and is the simplest fat that you want to clearly devour. Such fats are known as polyunsaturated fatty acids and monounsaturated fats, and not like saturated fat they remain in liquid shape at room temperature.

The zero.33 form of fats is trans-fat or trans-fatty acid. Tran-fat is a bad fat and have to be avoided the least bit charges. This form of fats is uncommon in nature and fashioned artificially whilst oil goes via a way referred to as hydrogenation, which essentially method to cope with with hydrogen.

Let's now take a look at every of these fats in a hint more detail.

1.Three.1 Saturated Fat

A excessive intake of saturated fats increases your ldl ldl cholesterol level and that in turn can make a contribution to excessive blood pressure, coronary coronary heart infection, and stroke.

Try now not to include any more than 10% saturated fats into your diet regime on the maximum. Any extra than 10% and the harms outweigh the blessings.

Here are 10 products in which you can generally find out saturated fat:

1.   Animal Fats

2.   Butter

3.   Cheese

4.   Chocolate

5.   Coconut

6.   Cream (heavy, whipping)

7.   Fish Oils

8.   Hydrogenated Oils

nine.   Nuts & seeds

10.   Processed Meats

On a facet be conscious, I could probably endorse you to in no way eat any horrific snacks within the the front of your teach before a recreation or exercising.

Believe me as soon as I say, a coach may get very disenchanted if he sees you disrespecting your body through chewing on any ingredients which can be dangerous to health.

He may additionally additionally moreover even positioned you on the bench simply to educate you a lesson. I even have visible this arise on severa sports through the years.

1.3.2 Unsaturated Fats

Whenever feasible, typically select out unsaturated fat over saturated fat. In assessment to saturated fat, this form of fat will genuinely decrease your "awful" LDL levels of cholesterol and moreover assist you to burn off more body weight.

Good resources of unsaturated fat in oils embody:

Olive oil

Rapeseed oil

Safflower oil (to name simply 3)

Polyunsaturated fats is a kind of unsaturated fat this is specifically useful to heart health. Good property of polyunsaturated fats embody

Butternuts

Cashew nuts

Herrings

Mackerel

Salmon

Sardines

Sunflower seeds

Trout

Tuna

Walnuts

Monounsaturated fat are every other sort of unsaturated fats. It is commonly decided in plant-based totally additives, but can also be located in some meat and dairy merchandise too.

Oils that encompass monounsaturated fats are normally liquid even as saved at room temperature, however they will begin to expose sturdy at the equal time as chilled under room temperature.

Good belongings of monounsaturated fats embody

Butter

Cheese (Parmesan cheese, Cheshire cheese, Cream cheese)

Dark chocolate

Eggs

Fish

Fruits (excessive fat) which includes olives and avocados

Nuts and seeds (numerous)

Red meats

Vegetable oils

My private preferred deliver for unsaturated fat is cashew nuts. They are fantastically moreish and I love to apply them in my cooking.

The fundamental disadvantage with those nuts is that I often consume too many (it is a prone aspect of mine). This forces me to work extra hard inside the route of exercise periods just so I can burn off the greater energy.

If you need nuts and moreover discover it hard to save you eating them once you begin, then you need to be organized to work more difficult than the others to your institution so you avoid gaining unwanted kilos.

Chapter 2: Vitamins And Soccer

Although normal exercise, exceptional tool, and the functionality to play proper football are all critical requirements on your fundamental improvement as a participant, not one of the above manners very heaps if you are vitamins deficient.

Vitamins in truth do have an impact on each element of your capability to play appropriate football, from the first-rate of your eyesight to the fee of your crosses.

If you discover which you're now not developing as rapid as you would really like to, then a lack of nutrients can be your problem.

You're probable thinking precisely what vitamins an up-and-coming football participant must make sure are stepping into his weight loss program. I will list a number of the maximum critical vitamins in this bankruptcy.

These are the ones which you should simply realize approximately. I also can be bringing up how the ones vitamins can beautify your interest. Most importantly, I will display you techniques of getting extra of them for your every day healthy dietweight-reduction plan.

2.1.1 Vitamin A

Vitamin A is likely quality regarded for its impact on eyesight. Although it obtained't offer you with on the spot night time time time imaginative and prescient, growing your diet regime A consumption should have a substantial effect in your potential to peer in low slight conditions.

Not having enough nutrition A, as a substitute, can motive problems with imaginative and prescient that might compromise your ability to play football at your complete capability.

Vitamin A doesn't without a doubt have an effect on vision despite the fact that. This multi-motive nutrients also promotes healthful pores and skin, bones, and teeth.

Fortunately, food plan A may be determined in a whole lot of components, which incorporates eggs, meat, and dairy merchandise, as well as in yellow, orange and green flowers. Vitamin A is a fat soluble nutrients, which means that that your body can preserve it until it is wanted.

2.1.2 The B Vitamins

Have you ever wanted you had only a little extra jump in the doorstep? Well, likely the B nutrients can assist.

Once perception to be a single diet, the B vitamins at the moment are stated to be a set of nutrients which might be needed to convert oxygen and electricity into electricity, and for you that interprets to more oomph on the sphere.

B Vitamins also assist your body produce vital things which include protein and blood cells.

Without them, your frame sincerely may not be capable of make new cells.

Furthermore, a deficiency in B vitamins may even positioned you at a higher chance of growing most cancers and extraordinary continual illnesses.

If you become deficient in B nutrients, for a few element reason, you may discover yourself missing video video games and practices due to infection.

That's due to the truth individuals who don't get sufficient B vitamins no longer first-class have less strength normally, but they may be more vulnerable to not unusual infection than individuals who are not nutrients B poor.

There are simply eight superb B nutrients, however the fine records is that they will be frequently positioned within the identical meals. So imparting you encompass those kinds of food into your each day diet regime, then there can be no motive on the way to turn out to be negative in weight loss plan B.

If you're in need of that kick of electricity that simplest B nutrients can provide you with, you then want to ensure you have become sufficient of the following styles of food onto your plate at mealtimes:

Whole grains

Seafood

Meats

Eggs

Legumes

Molasses

Leafy inexperienced vegetables.

Many sports activities activities and power liquids are also fortified with this energy-yielding organization of vitamins. Whether you are a carnivore or a vegetarian, it's now not difficult to find elements which containing weight loss program B.

Point to notice: Because the B nutrients are water soluble, it approach your body cannot keep them like it can fats soluble nutrients. Because of this, you need to encompass elements significant in weight loss program B into your "daily" weight loss plan.

2.1.Three Vitamin C

Are your accidents taking a piece too extended to heal, or are you bored stiff with catching each little malicious program that is going spherical?

If you answered sure to any of the above, then you definately definately are likely in need of some diet C.

It's tough to overstate the useful consequences of this water soluble food plan as it actually is important for assisting accurate fitness.

Vitamin C plays some of roles inner your frame, from stimulating the immune gadget to assisting wounds heal brief. It can also assist to fend off terminal illnesses like maximum cancers, thru manner of appearing as an antioxidant.

People who don't collect an terrific enough amount of this essential nutrients can come to be with the infamous scurvy ailment; a sickness which ends up in enamel loss and a breakdown of the body's connective tissue.

Many humans swear by the blessings of getting a hint vitamins C decorate at the number one symptoms of contamination.

Some of the additives which may be wealthy in weight loss program C content material cloth additionally will be predisposed to be acidic.

Here is a shortlist of some meals containing nutrients C:

Liver

Broccoli

Citrus stop cease result

Tomatoes

Berries

Tropical culmination (maximum)

As you could see, which consist of healthy dietweight-reduction plan C in your every day eating regimen is not only a healthful desire, but a scrumptious one as properly.

2.1.Four Vitamin D

If you need to have the strong bones wanted for taking walks and kicking, and bones which are resilient to difficult tackles, you then definately need to make sure you have become sufficient nutrition D for your food plan.

This fats-soluble nutrients is vital for each the development and the preservation of sturdy healthful bones. Vitamin D aids your potential to assume surely and additionally permits to decrease excessive blood stress.

Vitamin D can get into our gadget three techniques. It can be made inside the pores and pores and pores and skin from publicity to daytime, it could be consumed through certain food, and it is able to enter our frame in the form of dietary supplements, the latter usually being a completely ultimate lodge.

A right deliver of diet D can be had from the subsequent meals:

Beef liver

Cheese

Dairy merchandise

Egg yolks

Fatty fish

Fish oils

Mushrooms

Processed grains

2.1.Five Vitamin E

Most football game enthusiasts go through an entire lot of wear and tear and tear in the course of the direction of a sport. This makes diet E especially important because of its feature in mobile healing. It acts as an antioxidant, defensive mobile membranes.

This fats-soluble nutrition moreover permits to form the red blood cells which may be needed to supply oxygen spherical inside the blood. Without nutrition E on your system you received't be on the sector for too prolonged.

Vitamin E may be placed in lots of forms of food sources alongside aspect:

Avocados

Nuts

Seeds

Vegetable oils

Whole grains

This is the one fat-soluble antioxidant if you need to make you healthier, quicker, and greater wholesome.

2.1.6 Vitamin K

Vitamin K is a totally crucial vitamins due to the fact the frame desires it for its blood-clotting feature. This makes it a important nutrient for soccer gamers, and clearly people everywhere, however mainly in sports activities sports because it in reality is wherein nasty cuts and bleeding are much more likely to arise, greater regularly.

Vitamin K isn't handiest beneficial for its characteristic in blood clotting. It has unique critical roles as properly, like constructing sturdy bones and preventing coronary coronary heart disorder to call certainly , but there are a few precise crucial bodily techniques that it performs a detail in too.

Whichever way you study it, this fats-soluble nutrient is important in your sport, and so that you need to preserve nutrition K to your tool through way of ingesting the proper components. There are severa meals which might be right belongings of vitamins K, which include:

Dairy products

Leafy inexperienced veggies

Meats

Vegetable oils

All of the above ingredients, and some others except, provide sufficient food plan K so you can recover from the cuts and scrapes that necessarily come about in the game of soccer.

OK, that concludes our brief check the maximum essential nutrients. As you could see, taking nutrients through inclusive of meals into your weight-reduction plan which encompass enough portions of every have to make a large difference in your capability to play wonderful football.

It's no longer hard to get all of the vitamins you want from food, however it's far vital to realise which substances carries what vitamins, and now you do.

2.2 Minerals

There is a lot of communicate presently about minerals and the function they play in a healthful and active lifestyles. But paying attention to approximately the significance of minerals from professional nutritionists does no longer inform us masses extra than they may be vital!

Such one-liners are obviously scant on statistics and that is why many human beings although have unanswered questions on the proper function minerals play in our bodies. We want to understand greater!

As a football player, you have to probably apprehend a few factor apart from the fact that minerals are "suitable for you" so that you can use them to promote better health and fitness stages.

For this, you may need to understand precisely what minerals do to your body, specifically, and most significantly, can they will let you grow to be a higher player than if you have been say mineral deficient? In unique terms, is this a few element clearly well worth the trouble of reading approximately?

In short, positive it's miles.

Knowing the 'mineral basics' is treasured information for you as a sports sports man or woman.

OK, permit's start to look at minerals in a touch more detail.

2.2.1 What are minerals?

Minerals are also referred to as micronutrients. They are essential organisms desired throughout our entire lifestyles, in small portions. Minerals at the whole orchestrate diverse physical capabilities which may be vital for healthful living.

Because our our bodies do no longer make those minerals without a doubt, we want to consequently get them from our food plan or from severa supplements.

Although they make up tons less than four percent of the human body, a variety of our most essential techniques would possibly no longer be capable of characteristic without important minerals.

There are numerous minerals that everyone need of their food plan, specifically:

Potassium

Sodium

Calcium

Phosphorus

Magnesium

Zinc

Iron

Iodine

Manganese

2.2.2 Why will we want minerals without a doubt?

Although there are various certainly one in all a type minerals, most of them have a commonplace denominator. They are the constructing blocks of your body's cells; they may be liable for regulating first-rate chemical reactions and methods.

Some minerals, along with calcium and manganese, help to assemble healthful bones. Others, like iron, useful resource the frame in producing wholesome blood cells.

Each of the minerals performs a extremely good however important role, all supporting to construct and maintain a robust and healthful you.

The more wholesome you're everyday, the extra capable you becomes as a football participant. Having a nicely-nourished frame continually offers you with the considered necessary electricity and power had to compete and take part as a precious member of your group.

2.2.Three How do minerals have an effect on soccer game enthusiasts?

It is vital that everybody, in particular football gamers, get adequate portions of all the vital minerals, after which make certain they hold the ones tiers always.

Your body is being taxed to extremes on every occasion you are taking component in a opposition or a hard training consultation. You most possibly depart each activity now not genuinely with a heavy dose of fatigue, however furthermore with some bumps, bruises, and scrapes further.

It's critical that you are able to repair your fatigued muscle mass as quick as possible, however you furthermore mght want to maintain constructing on the stamina and electricity you've got already were given so that you can play even higher subsequent time. Don't neglect approximately, until you reach your pinnacle, there may be always room for upgrades.

Imagine now not being capable of heal short from a minor scrape, or maybe upward thrust up from a mild fall as it's knocked the stuffing out of you. This is what the fact looks like with out an adequate quantity of minerals to your system.

It's easy to peer how getting sufficient minerals, or no longer getting enough minerals, ought to make all the difference for your activity.

Making wonderful you've got were given a healthful food plan, one which incorporates all the important vitamins and minerals, prepares you for achievement on and off the arena.

When a body is properly-nourished and energized it makes you enjoy able to doing some thing, and that in flip has a wonderful effect on the way you enjoy mentally as properly. In other terms, it's far all correct.

2.2.Four Sodium and potassium

There are mineral sorts that play a vital position on your frame during your exercise and video games, especially sodium and potassium.

These minerals are what is known as electrolytes, or salts in simple English. They input and exit your muscle cells all through muscular contraction and relaxation.

Electrolytes stay inside the blood, and different body fluids, and convey an electric powered price. They furthermore have an effect on the quantity of water there is for your body at any given time, the acidity of your blood known as (pH), and your muscle function, along aspect a few special essential techniques.

When you're training or gambling video games, a huge quantity of these electrolytes are out of vicinity via your sweat.

When this takes region, there may be an imbalance to your frame. You may additionally additionally have visible salt earrings in your garments after a exercise. The lack of these salts may be dangerous if they will be no longer replenished.

You can often electrolytes marketed at the labels of numerous sports sports activities drinks (make certain to observe the content material fabric fabric label to make certain), so consuming those earlier than, in the course of and after your exercising and video video games is probably some detail you need to investigate. Electrolytes additionally can be observed in some power bars too.

However, in case you favor to bypass sugary sports activities sports beverages then nutrient-wealthy end end end result, vegetables, dairy, and entire grains are the herbal way to inventory up on, and update minerals out of place within the course of lively interest.

In truth, many expert gamers could likely choose to consume a salty soup or first-rate elements containing electrolytes as their pre-pastime meal.

2.2.Five Calcium

So, why do you want calcium?

Well, you possibly do not forget your parents telling you as a piece teenager which you want to drink plenty of milk because it's suitable in your enamel, nails and bones, and that it's miles going that will help you to expand stronger. They had been now not incorrect.

Milk is a truely exceptional deliver of calcium together with yogurt, and cheese too, however some types are higher than others.

Dairy is honestly the high-quality recognize supply of calcium however isn't the simplest meals type to include this critical nutrient (see list beneath).

To enhance your calcium intake and feature your opponents bouncing off your sturdy frame in the course of a sport, make certain to include some or all the following substances into you regular food plan:

Low Fat Cheese

Low Fat Yogurts

Non Fat or 1% Milk

Non-every day additives encompass:

Cereals

Fruits (diverse)

Leafy vegetables

Legumes

Seafood

Numerous food and drink also are fortified with the mineral, however normally select the greater herbal assets whenever viable.

Remember this: in case you're not getting sufficient calcium on your diet, then your body will take what it dreams from your bones. It has to do this to ensure normal cell feature.

But the trouble with taking calcium out of your bones on a everyday basis is that it may cause weakened bones, and also you in truth do no longer need that to take area.

So make certain you get all the calcium your frame needs thru which consist of calcium-rich substances into your everyday food plan.

2.2.6 Iron

Iron works as a transporter of oxygen within the course of your body. If you don't get enough of it inside the course of exercising and video video games, the consequences are immediately.

If your iron tiers are low you then definately virtually'll get worn-out pretty rapid. In distinct phrases, your general typical performance on the world will visit pot notably.

To save you iron deficiency from going on you could want to encompass iron-rich meals into your regular meals.

Don't worry, those of you who already eat balanced food will already be doing this, that means you may not need to regulate your food plan very lots, if in any respect (see listing below).

Chapter 3: Diets

Ask any professional soccer player and he's going to surly will let you know of the significance of ingesting right. Consuming a carefully-attuned weight loss plan, together with ingesting masses of fluids, is vital to any football participant's customary performance on the field.

three.1 The Atkins Diet?

If you are a football player you ought to attempt to keep away from the Atkins food plan and particular Atkins-kind diets the least bit expenses. This is due to the fact the Atkins diet regime calls for that you consume plenty of protein at the same time as warding off maximum carbohydrates.

Without a superb consumption of exquisite carbohydrates, you'll not be able to perform at height-degrees on the sphere. This is due to the truth carbohydrates offer your important supply of fuel while operating towards or playing soccer.

Before each schooling session and endeavor you need to already be stocked-up on unique-first-rate carbs. This will make certain that you can play at your complete capacity because the carbs provide you with the power you want.

When you've got tremendous electricity stages you could play with electricity, expertise, and preserve your stamina for the duration of the game.

The nearly carb-loose Atkins healthy eating plan and notable low-carb ingesting plans, can significantly and detrimentally have an effect for your simple ordinary overall performance.

A stable football weight loss plan need to encompass at least forty five% carbohydrates, with 25% proteins and 30% fats. Any important variation to the above will see a drop for your typical overall performance. It sincerely is as smooth as that.

This technique you need to make carbohydrates your essential meals deliver, and simply the foundation of your food plan. Quality, staple carbs encompass pasta, rice, and potatoes.

However, it is no longer pretty a good buy the carbs. The most essential problem right right here is stability, so you have to now not dismiss the importance of proteins and fat in the healthy eating plan either. You simply need to adjust how an entire lot you eat of each.

Protein is crucial for a balanced eating regimen. It not handiest permits to build robust bones and muscle tissues, but it moreover aids in the frame-repair method after strenuous video video video games and accidents.

Fat is likewise vital for desired health and properly being. It strengthens your immune machine and allows guard in opposition to contamination.

Good fat may be placed in oily and fatty fish. These are a wealthy supply of omega-3 fatty acids, that is a sort of fats that is exceptional for fitness.

It may be futile attempting to find to play regular football on an Atkins-style eating regimen. Sooner, in desire to later, you may find out your self having to exchange again to a greater traditional food plan.

In brief, the absence of carbohydrates for your meals could have a very bad impact on your ability to play at your remarkable.

I am not saying that the Atkins weight loss program, or a few different low-carb fashion diet regime, is awful in famous. In truth, it's miles very useful for individuals who want to shed kilos fast for fitness reasons, and in all likelihood for others who do not participate in speedy, physical sporting sports activities.

However, the Atkins diet plan is not a soccer weight-reduction plan as it will not provide you with the critical fuel to practice, play, and get higher.

3.2 Organic Diet

Organic diets are an exceptional way to bring together and keep right fitness and fitness. Before I describe how an natural weight loss plan can do that, I will first provide an cause in the back of precisely what an natural diet surely is.

Many think of the word 'herbal' to intend uncooked-meals. This isn't the case, but. The time period herbal refers to meals that has been grown the usage of traditional farming techniques, that is, with out using risky chemical sellers.

In one of a kind phrases, a return to number one farming techniques; practices that have been in place lengthy earlier than those varieties of insecticides, fungicides and herbicides have emerge as the norm; loads of which might be said to poison the earth.

The very last results of eating non-organic meals manner there can be commonly a capability risk to human fitness every time we consume devices grown the usage of modern-day agricultural techniques.

This is because of the truth the chemical substances from the sellers which can be used on crops are then ingested into the body. That can't be appropriate for human health, it absolutely can't be.

The cease result of in depth, modern-day farming has additionally meant that the soil has progressively become depleted of its herbal nutrients.

Nutrient-depleted soil way that the flora grown in it also are lacking in dietary fee in evaluation to flora grown in soil which is not nutrient poor, as is the case with an natural farm.

So uncooked food does not always advocate it's miles natural food. You may want to have raw-natural or raw non-organic food. Raw honestly method food which isn't always cooked or processed.

Eating uncooked, natural food is an extraordinary way of supplying your body with the right forms of nutrients, and without ingesting volatile pollutants within the method.

Raw meals, in favored, consists of many more manifestly-happening nutrients and minerals than food it really is cooked or processed, and especially uncooked-natural food.

These essential nutrients and minerals are what help the frame to characteristic resultseasily and gain resilience against disorder and injury.

And within the case wherein we do emerge as unwell or injured, the healthier our diet regime has been, the earlier we are probable to recover from any disorder.

Anyone seeking to acquire most fitness and fitness will combine an herbal weight-reduction plan with a regular consumption of fluids so that they remain in a hydrated state continually.

Water is the fantastic fluid you could drink, without exception, and first-rate of all is that clean consuming water it's miles with out trouble and freely to be had, in most western worldwide places, so make specific use of your faucet.

Under everyday occasions, you have to purpose for at least 10 massive (33cl) glasses of water each day to keep your hydration tiers. Most humans do not, thru the manner, an awful lot to their detriment.

Whenever parents begin to tire later inside the day, it is frequently due to the fact they may be experiencing the early stages of dehydration, and now not due to the fact they may be exhausted by using using their paintings or some physical interest.

Water also assists your frame in flushing out pollutants. Some of the uncooked food types you could consist of into your food plan (cucumber and watermelon as examples) may even depend as a part of your well-known fluid consumption.

Keeping to an natural diet plan, mixed with the consumption of loads of glowing-water, will offer your body with all that it needs to carry out at its maximum appropriate levels. It's a clean recipe for success.

3.Three Soccer Diet Example

A healthful diet full of terrific strength-rich elements will permit your normal usual performance-levels to boom exponentially. Eating terrible elements, but, need to have the possibility impact.

A suitable food regimen for soccer game enthusiasts have to be carb-wealthy. What substances and what type of exactly may be adjusted slightly every time a sport and exercise consultation is nearing. Avoid dangerous processed factors, rapid elements, and snack factors including hamburgers or sweet.

As tasty and as tempting as the ones might be to you, definitely apprehend that they play no position inside the life of an up-and-coming, or already successful, soccer player, in particular earlier than a sport.

The following desk contains a balanced dietary plan that is appropriate for any soccer player:

Breakfast   Lunch Dinner

Milk (of a low-fats range)   Fish   (wealthy   in Omega 3 fatty acid) Chicken (skinless)

Pancakes   Pasta Lean meat

Potatoes   Bread (whole-meal). Multigrain bread is a long way advanced to white bread)
          Rice (brown or white)

Fruits Soups Vegetables

Yoghurt   Salad (with out dressing)

Chapter 4: Fluids

In this chapter you're approximately to discover the real significance of fluids, or extra specially, hydration. This is something that may really make or destroy your exercise.

4.1 Hydration

A activity of soccer exerts immoderate wishes at the body. One of the essential issue strategies of combatting the effects of those desires is to stay properly hydrated continually.

This involves the everyday intake of clean, healthy beverages, preferably water, to replace the fluids you lose via perspiration inside the direction of the sport.

Indeed, as your frame heats up, it starts offevolved to sweat profusely in its try to strive and funky you down. Just like a car engine requires water to prevent it from overheating, so too does the human body.

It isn't always most effective at some point of fits that you'll need to maintain in mind to live hydrated. Any workout video video games, schooling classes, and intervals of exercise need to all be performed at the same time as being sufficiently hydrated.

In a nutshell, in case you're now not well hydrated then you truly might not be capable of carry out at your first-rate and nor will you experience in top circumstance.

Hydration suggestions:

Always quench your thirst. In truth, you must not even wait until you are thirsty in advance than you drink.

Milk may be below the have an effect on of alcohol now and again as a water replacement. Aim for the skimmed or semi-skimmed variety.

The occasional sports sports drink can also depend as a water substitute, despite the fact that be careful of those. Most sports activities sports activities drinks are loaded with extra sugar and want to be ate up in moderation or after strenuous bouts of bodily hobby. If you hold appropriate, everyday hydration tiers, then there must be no need to consume sports activities activities sports beverages to top off loss fluids under regular conditions.

Avoid all sodas and any carbonated beverages that include heaps of sugar, additives, and preservatives.

Drinks containing caffeine (tea, espresso, and cola) make you pee more regularly and therefore counteract the hydration gadget. Drink such liquids cautiously and keep away from them altogether on recreation days.

four.2 Dehydration

Dehydration is the term used to provide an cause of the usa that your frame enters while you do now not have the correct portions of fluid in your machine.

You are losing precious fluids all of the time, on the identical time as you sweat, urinate, vomit, have diarrhea, or perhaps at the same time as you breathe. If you do no longer often update the out of place water out of your frame, then you may rapid start to undergo the results of early dehydration.

For football gamers, dehydration is a particularly common hassle in the path of video games, especially the ones which can be accomplished underneath a heat sun, wherein profuse sweating and heavy respiration reasons big water loss in a reasonably quick region of time.

I realize from revel in that many novice gamers absolutely don't address board sufficient water in the route of video games; some thing that serves to their drawback.

Here are the five primary signs of early dehydration:

1.   Feeling very thirsty

2.   Feeling lightheaded

3.   A quickened heartbeat

4.   Dryness across the mouth and lips

five. Infrequent urination and/or dark coloured and strong-smelling urine

4.Three Water

Water is highly undervalued as a difficulty of an first rate football eating regimen amongst amateurs.

Most expert players select to drink water in area of sugary sports activities sports drinks, not because of the fact they choose the flavor of water, it truely is quite flavorless except, however because of the fact they recognize that it is through an extended way the incredible fluid for keeping the body in a hydrated country.

Sports or caffeine-based absolutely liquids provide an super energy improve but will no longer replenish your fluids in the same way that water will. They may also additionally furthermore even contribute to dehydration whilst below the influence of alcohol in huge portions.

Providing you hold a ordinary regime wherein you by no means allow your self to become dehydrated, then water is your brilliant choice of fluid.

Not only will your body stay hydrated, however you'll you moreover mght enjoy more healthful and stronger and consequently get to decorate your performance on the world due to this.

Another problem really worth bringing up is that dehydrated muscle mass are more likely to cramp-up and fatigue quicker than muscle companies which is probably hydrated and functioning usually.

The best hydration advice is as a way to in no way allow yourself to get thirsty inside the first region. If you experience thirsty within the course of a activity or a workout consultation, specially fast after the begin, then it's far maximum in all likelihood too past due to do masses about it.

Even in case you down a bucketful of water, it is not going to help masses. If a few difficulty, it will probably stop you similarly due to the huge quantity of water that now lies intently in your stomach.

Preempt your thirst thru way of drinking small quantities at normal periods. This is the great manner to completely stave off dehydration and to save you the above scenario ever happening to you.

It is certainly useful to hold a sports sports bottle complete of water with you at all times. This manner, you can keep your hydration while no longer having to search for a tap or a store that sells bottled water each time you're out and about.

I've definitely made this into a healthy dependancy. What because of this is if I do take region to head away the house without my water, I by no means get quite some steps away earlier than I be conscious it is lacking.

I truly like to freeze my water in a unmarried day due to the fact this way it is saved excellent and refreshingly bloodless at some level within the day.

As said in advance inside the monetary catastrophe, an exquisite way of telling whether or not your frame is turning into dehydrated or now not is through the shade of your urine.

So subsequent time you visit the relaxation room recall to test the color of your pee. Healthy urine contains materials which offer it its mild yellow tint.

If your urine is darkish orange it technique the ones materials are undiluted, and that indicates which you within the meanwhile are inside the early degrees of dehydration. The darker it's far, the extra you'll need to drink that allows you to fill up misplaced fluids.

four.Three.1 How a lot is sufficient?

There is an unofficial fashionable while speakme approximately the amount of water you should devour each day.

In fact, there can be masses confusion in the scientific community about hydration and simply how a amazing deal fluid we should drink on not unusual, beneath diverse conditions.

Let's not overlook too, that some humans perspire masses more than others, and glaringly they come to be dehydrated quicker as a end result.

The unofficial preferred recommends that we drink at the least 8-10 complete glasses (33cl) of water regular with day, underneath normal situations.

However, whilst you're collaborating in football schooling or video video games, this stylish obviously is going out of the window because those conditions are an extended manner from normal.

The extra you exert your self, the greater water you may need to eat to replenish those lost fluids, and as you apprehend, there is a lot of physical exertion taking region on a soccer location.

The minimal amount of water you want to likely drink at some point of a 24 hour length want to be no a lot less than three liters.

You will want to drink loads of water in advance than a sport so you're properly hydrated at kickoff. It's critical to drink water at some point of the sport as well due to the fact you want to hold your hydration tiers.

You furthermore want to keep ingesting water at everyday durations after the very last whistle has blown.

It is suggested which you drink 1-2 liters approximately   hours before your game. Whether it's miles one or liters is predicated upon on your hydration degree earlier than the 2 hours preceding to kickoff.

During the game, you need to attempt to consume about 7-10 oz.Each fifteen to twenty mins whenever possible.

four.Three.2 Improved common performance

You will now not beautify your ball abilities simply by using ingesting water constant with se. However, your trendy ordinary overall performance on the world can be plenty better than when you have been to play in a greater dehydrated country. That is a reality.

Improved performance method every physical and mentally. You will, as an instance, be capable of run and paintings more difficult for longer durations with out tiring.

Furthermore, your interest also can be better, which makes you more alert normally, therefore minimizing the functionality for errors.

4.Three.Three Not enough water

If your body is brief on water then you definitely definately genuinely'll begin to dehydrate quite rapid. That approach you can start to sense vulnerable and dizzy as a consequence, mainly in case you maintain pushing yourself tough at the same time as in this kingdom.

If you do begin to feel plenty much less than ordinary, then you definately virtually need to take without delay movement. Ignoring the symptoms and signs and symptoms and signs might also moreover need to result in you truly fainting or collapsing; some detail that is not all that unusual among newbie gamers.

The amount of water you devour before, within the path of, and after a hobby depends in large part at the weather. During heat summer time days you may glaringly need to consume greater water than you'll do whilst playing in cold climate.

4.Four Sports Drinks

We've already touched lightly with regards to sports activities activities drinks and now we are going to have a look at them a chunk more carefully.

Today, we're continuously bombarded with commercials at the tv at the internet and in print, all of which urge us to consume their candy and colourful sports activities sports beverages, convincing us, or searching to influence us, that those all-easy, all-hydrating drinks are the super invention considering sliced bread.

But are they, genuinely?

Quite frequently, a relied on movie star is the face of the product, suggesting which you could additionally revel in or gain what they revel in or reap as a right away give up end result of ingesting something sports sports sports activities drink it's miles they may be selling.

So what are those miracle products?

What exactly makes a drink a sports sports activities drink?

Who desires them?

And do they clearly make a difference?

OK, permit's have a look at every of those questions in flip.

4.Four.1 What is a sports drink?

A sports drink is supposed to help athletes, and other lively humans, recover quick from immoderate levels of interest. They provide extra than your not unusual beverage because of the fact they do extra than in truth pinnacle off misplaced fluids.

As nicely as collectively with salts and sugars, which assist to quick hydrate a dehydrated body, sports activities activities beverages also encompass various vitamins.

These nutrients help to repair the frame's electrolyte stability. The liquid carbohydrates contained inside those drinks provide a far needed strength decorate to an otherwise tired athlete.

Sports drinks aren't most effective greater healthy than many different sorts of beverages offered in excessive-road refrigerators, but they may be furthermore tastier too, and therefore more palatable than simple water.

The fitness element, mixed with tremendous flavors, has made sports activities sports liquids a fave among athletes from each recreation.

But are they certainly desired?

The method to that is no, not genuinely, no longer if you can maintain your hydration levels with natural water consumption, that is typically the satisfactory desire. And sports activities activities sports drinks should clearly not replace your every day water consumption.

4.Four.2 Do soccer gamers need sports activities sports beverages?

In a few instances, sports sports drinks may be very useful to soccer game enthusiasts, in particular whilst gambling difficult in a excessive-tempo interest for an prolonged time frame under a warm summer time sun. In situations like this you'll be sweating excessively, dropping not genuinely fluids, however furthermore electrolytes.

So every so often it is higher for soccer gamers to get a bit electricity increase from sports activities liquids, in particular even as playing underneath conditions like the one noted above.

Replacing fluid without addressing the dearth of minerals can bring about a risky scenario called water intoxication.

Drinking a sports sports drink replaces no longer in reality the fluids out of place, but the electrolytes as properly. Despite the apparent blessings of consuming sports sports activities beverages, there is, nonetheless, a stability that wants to be struck right proper here.

So the key's getting to know your personal body properly, and understand the manner to high-quality to maintain its hydration levels. This way, you becomes greater worried in prevention than you will be treatment, this is a far better manner to be.

4.Four.Three Making your non-public sports sports drinks

Sports beverages sold in plastic bottles may be every pricey and lousy for the surroundings. For this motive, many amateur football gamers absolutely drink water alternatively.

However, consuming high-quality water can, on events, bring about an electrolyte imbalance, especially if the frame isn't always maintained properly with the aid of the use of way of precise weight loss program.

Anyone who does have an electrolyte imbalance, even a mild one, cannot assume to carry out as well as they would do inside the occasion that they didn't have this imbalance.

There is an opportunity to the pricey and fancy-packaged sports activities activities beverages sold in high avenue stores, and it comes within the shape of a powder.

These powdered options are genuinely added to water then stirred. That's it. You now have a less pricey, but notwithstanding the reality that clearly as actual, selfmade sports activities activities drink made from a primary additives.

If you would like to have a chunk greater manage in making your very very own sports sports sports drinks from powders, then there are several commercially available manufacturers which can be famous among football gamers. These powders are available a giant form of flavors so it need to be clean enough to discover some element you enjoy.

Note that the ones powdered drinks will all variety pretty regular with their carbohydrate (CHO) and electrolyte content material cloth, along with the addition of various additives.

This is glaringly a far less expensive opportunity than the bottled kinds.

However, if you really want to hold the prices right down and feature entire control over each the contents and the flavor, then why no longer make your non-public sports beverages from scratch?

This is a completely clean technique in which all you need are some easy substances from throughout the kitchen, especially fruit squash or juice, sugar, salt, and water.

With a chunk of imagination you currently have a low-fee sports activities sports drink that meets all of your rehydration needs, and additionally one that tastes exactly the manner you need it to taste.

So as you can see, getting the electrolytes you need to fill up lost body fluids doesn't need to be steeply-priced, tough, or awful for the planet. A quick are attempting to find on-line will reveal a plethora of selfmade recipes so you can try at your entertainment.

four.Five Alternative Hydration

During a aggressive soccer exercise, strength and water is worn-out from the body at an alarming fee. While there can be no magic drink to present you your energy lower lower back in nanoseconds, you can nevertheless take concrete steps to rehydrate your self in the quickest way possible.

While water and sports sports activities liquids are usually considered the splendid picks for hydration, there are numerous other options that can contribute toward giving your body the water it wishes.

These supplementary alternatives are numerous meals items. They now not excellent make a contribution in your water consumption, however moreover they provide you with a few welcome range from consuming handiest beverages:

Watermelon: Not best is that this fruit 90 percent water, but it also gives a great range of vitamins and nutrients too, all of which assist you to stay in top shape. The wonderful way to hold watermelon to the sphere is to throw some cold watermelon cubes in a thermos or cooler wherein they may be saved excellent and chilled.

Grapes: These actually have a excessive percent of water content material material and include a few very key nutrients. They also are a neat, portable, mess-unfastened snack which could both be saved cool in a cooler or eaten at room temperature.

Jell-O: Most people comprehend that gelatin is almost truely water, however few recollect it in terms of a rehydration preference. You can store a gelatin combo in a thermos or a cooler, similar to watermelon. To hydrate powdered gelatin, honestly sprinkle it in cold water and allow it take a seat for five -10 minutes earlier than consuming (it takes as a minimum that long to dissolve in cool water). Just make sure to maintain it cool, or it is able to exchange into gelatin water, which is not something you may need to devour as it clearly is a shape of sticky liquid.

Cucumbers: Cucumbers are yet another natural food that may be a brilliant source of water. In truth, a cucumber is spherical 90 percentage water. Not handiest are the cucumber peels wealthy in insoluble fiber, which allows to hold a healthy digestive machine, however those nourishing snacks furthermore encompass diet A and food plan C. Try to preserve your cucumbers cool due to the fact they will be a crunchier, greater easy snack while chilled.

Below are some horrible hydration alternatives in drink form, alongside facet the motives why they may be not first rate alternatives. Despite this truth, some dad and mom although pick out them as their hydration answer, even though they in all likelihood won't do for a good deal longer within the occasion that they observe this listing.

Caffeinated drinks: Caffeine in reality dehydrates because of its diuretic effect (makes you pee extra regularly). Therefore, regardless of the reality that caffeine liquids are despite the fact that fluids, they contribute in the direction of dehydration, no longer hydration.

High sugar juices: Fructose, the sugar actually present in fruits, simply slows down the device that the body goes thru at the identical time as absorbing water. Drinking it can truly make you feel unwell because of the fact the fluid will slosh round uncomfortably because it waits to be absorbed.

Carbonated liquids: These can purpose bloating and make you too uncomfortable to play at your whole functionality. Further, nearly all of those beverages encompass phosphoric acid in the elements, something which reduces calcium inside the bones.

Chapter 5: Game Food

No this isn't always a side chapter on wild animals and birds (hobby) which might be hunted and eaten, but a economic catastrophe on football vitamins.

Here I will give an reason for the pleasant sorts of meals to consume in advance than, throughout and after a recreation. We may additionally actually have a check what you should consume whilst gambling video games in the morning or late night time.

five.1 The morning sport

I don't apprehend approximately you, but for my part I used to hate early morning games. The purpose for this grow to be that I typically felt a lack of strength at that element of day.

Heck, I couldn't even take part in the warmup with out searching for to relaxation midway via.

However, this became all in advance than I discovered the call of the game within the once more of ingesting the right forms of food. These are meals that prepare you particularly for early morning hobby.

The meals inside the desk below will price your frame with lots of a whole lot desired electricity. Once you begin to consume components from this list you may be able to carry out in the early morning while not having to pull your toes every step of the manner.

The days of getting tired simply 10 mins after the beginning whistle is blown turns into a issue of the beyond. There is probably no extra hoping all of it ends quickly simply so you can circulate slowly decrease back home and take a high-quality prolonged nap.

For this alteration to appear, you will want to realise a manner to eat the proper form of gasoline. These components will give you the energy you need for acting at your awesome within the ones early morning video video games of soccer.

Below is a table listing the early morning superfoods, which incorporates items to keep away from (showed in the ultimate column).

Meal	Drinks	Dessert	Avoid
Bagels	Apple Juice	Fruit Bar	1st Baron Beaverbrook
Oatmeal	Orange Juice	Fruit	Sausage
Bread	Vegetable Juice Butter	Raisins	
Yogurt	Hot chocolate	Banana	All Fried materials.

five.2 Evening enterprise

Like many soccer gamers, I pick to play video video games within the night. This is because I typically experience extra prepared at that issue of day. It is likewise an awful lot less complex to set up food because of the fact I don't need to pressure about time even as getting prepared and cooking meals later inside the day.

In the table beneath I actually have listed a few examples of the elements that I devour in guidance for midnight video video games, inclusive of gadgets to avoid (established within the final column).

The version and combination of meals that may be had from this listing is restrained only thru your imagination.

Meal	Drinks	Dessert	Avoid
Spaghetti	Orange Juice	Cheese Sugar	
Chicken & Salad	Vegetable Popcorn	Chocolate	Juice
Salad	Water	Fruit	Chips
Fish & Potatoes	Fruit Juice Tacos		Pretzels

5.Three Post-Game

The primary cause for eating food and beverage immediately after a exercise session or undertaking is to rehydrate your frame and top off your muscle tissues with new electricity.

The table under offers you recommendations on what to consume put up-in shape that lets in you to get the most advantage, and also includes gadgets to keep away from (proven in the last column).

My favourite mixture is to consume a fruit salad, drink masses of water (despite the reality that not in a unmarried move), and quit off with a tasty energy bar.

Sometimes it can be pretty hard to devour some thing virtually 30-60 minutes after a endeavor is over. The purpose for this is due to the fact the difficult bodily exertion expended in a energetic sport of football can, in some human beings, suppress appetite.

If you have got that "I'm genuinely not hungry" feeling, then attempt to as a minimum consume a protein bar, multiple bananas, or a small sandwich made with white bread.

Here's the table of recommended meals devices amazing fed on right now after a recreation or workout consultation.

Meal	Drinks	Dessert	Avoid	
Honey	Energy Drinks		Fruit Bars	Sir Francis Beaverbrook
Bagel	Water	Fruit	Sausage	
Banana	Lemonade		Raisins	
	Butter			
Jams	Vegetable Juice		Bars	Fried Foods

Chapter 6: Myths, Tips And Maximum Performance

There are hundreds of fake truths circulating about football diets nowadays. These may be very perplexing to quite a few human beings, specially whilst you're new to the arena of vitamins.

There will constantly be a few human beings who've in no manner even glanced at a soccer vitamins e-book but experience licensed to offer recommendation on what ought to and have to not be eaten as part of a football participant's weight loss plan.

This is facts that's pretty regularly picked up and handed on with the aid of using others who're similarly unauthorized on the challenge and consequently devices a terrible precedent.

6.1 Common myths

To help you navigate this minefield of facts, and extra importantly the incorrect information it honestly is available, I will debunk a number of the greater common myths related to football nutrients, and observe how numerous meals have an impact on commonplace overall performance on the sphere.

6.1.1 Your normal overall performance is not laid low with what you eat.

This is complete and utter nonsense and one fable that you should dismiss sincerely. Your normal overall performance is very a whole lot inspired with the beneficial resource of what you eat.

The better the nutritional fine of the meals you consume, the better your performances may be. It absolutely is as clean as that.

You simply can't gorge on a slice of fudge cake a few hours in advance than a hobby and anticipate to be on pinnacle form. It can be hard to withstand, however you want to live away from this type of dangerous snacking, at the least on endeavor days, in particular if you're excessive approximately growing as a player.

6.1.2 What you eat after a sport doesn't have an effect on your healing.

Every newbie football participant has feasted on some of the worst viable positioned up-in form additives ever, especially chips, sodas, and chocolate bars.

This kind of junk scoffing need to be prevented the least bit charges. Intelligent put up-healthy eating will embody end result, strength bars, and lots of water (see desk above for a listing of endorsed placed up-undertaking meals gadgets).

A enough amount of properly-great carbohydrates is needed after a fit to assist your body get better properly. Sugary, salty, processed snacks surely cannot do that for you.

6.1.3 It doesn't depend quantity in case you consume one, or five hours earlier than a recreation.

Oh positive it does.

You need to make sure you go away as a minimum four hours among eating and kick-off time.

In some instances, like early morning games as an example, you can lessen this time to 3 hours, however surely no a first-rate deal a lot much less than that.

Your frame preferably desires at the least 4 hours to digest and method the food you devour.

One of the maximum energy-efficient pre-fit meals is spaghetti and meat sauce. The mixture of the sauce and the pasta gives you a meal this is every carb and protein-wealthy.

A easy meal like this may provide you with a big energy beautify so that it will permit you to closing the period of a exercise with out feeling fatigued half of manner thru.

6.1.Four Drinking or not ingesting water doesn't have an impact to your normal normal performance.

Anyone who buys into this fable have to try and play on the same time as they may be not properly hydrated and seen how they fare.

Of path, consuming exact enough amounts of water is vital on your success on the sector.

Not handiest have to you drink small quantities of water at set periods in advance than a recreation, but furthermore on the identical time as the game is going on, and after it has completed.

In other phrases, hydration is an ongoing workout (see financial disaster four for information).

A soccer membership must keep plenty of reachable water at the sidelines and at the back of the goals clearly so game enthusiasts can inventory-up on water reserves speedy and resultseasily for the duration of video video games.

Remember, your body is type of a automobile in as loads as with out gas, or the incorrect form of gas, it will both now not paintings or no longer perform as well as it should do. Proper food and clean ingesting water is top fee fuel for the human body.

So ensure you hold your water consumption excessive by using way of stepping into the dependancy of drinking as a minimum liters of the stuff within the hours critical as plenty as a enterprise or practice session.

6.2 Maximize your performance ranges

Performing at your height on the area technique more than truly putting in a hundred% try on the identical time as you are there. Being dedicated is important, however it is quality one a part of your common soccer fulfillment.

You need to additionally pay close attention to the finer information of your education off the arena in addition to giving your whole recognition while on it.

Indeed, football improvement is type of a small puzzle, which means there are numerous portions to it that all want to be positioned into area, within the proper order, earlier than the whole thing finally comes collectively.

If you have actually one piece left out of the puzzle, or positioned inside the incorrect place, the outcome is probably damaging in your everyday normal performance stages.

OK, permit us to now have a have a take a look at the ones clean, yet crucial portions of the "soccer achievement puzzle" in more detail.

Rest

Nutrition

Sleep

Focus

6.2.1 Sufficient relaxation

Before each activity or schooling consultation you want to make certain you have got had been given had sufficient relaxation in order that your body is virtually energized and organized for the pains earlier.

Therefore, it's miles essential that you do not get concerned in every other shape of bodily interest for twenty-4 hours in advance than kick-off.

As you rest you could pursue some thing that helps you to lighten up. That might be kicking again to take a look at TV, gambling video video video games, listening to tune, analyzing a e-book, or some thing else works for you.

It certainly does no longer rely range what it's miles so long as it'd not require physical exertion.

6.2.2 Quality Nutrition

The importance top notch nutrients can not be overstated. Consuming the proper types of food is vital for your soccer improvement and normal average performance.

Without precise enough nutrition, neither your body nor your thoughts can be capable of function at its maximum appropriate. In other phrases, your preferred overall performance can be inhibited to a few degree, relying on how undernourished you are at the time.

Again, we will use the automobile analogy to consider this. If I fill my vehicle with masses of top elegance fuel, it'll pass an prolonged manner, however if I handiest positioned a small amount in, and a substandard fuel at that, then it'll want refilling another time speedy afterward plus it's going to carry out poorly while it is walking.

Your frame is not any notable. Fill it with low incredible food and drinks (gasoline) and you may now not best speedy run out of electricity, but your commonplace performance might be below par too.

The essential shape of gas needed via your frame for playing a hit football is carbohydrates. This strength supply can be determined in factors like pasta, bread, potatoes, rice, and numerous end result.

It's critical to preserve in mind, however, that not all carbohydrates are a high-quality supply of gasoline for football players.

These are the "clean carbohydrates" and placed specifically in processed food like chips, sweet, and soda drinks.

None of those gadgets will bring you any lasting, fine energy as they encompass what is called empty electricity, this is, calories derived from materials which encompass no nutritional charge.

6.2.Three Enough Sleep

Ever participated in a game after a horrible night time's sleep? If you haven't, I can tell you from enjoy that it isn't a pleasing prevalence the least bit, in truth it could be torture.

To placed it actually, without at least eight hours of exceptional kip (the commonplace required via maximum people), then your frame will no longer be sufficiently rested for it to reap height overall performance, or clearly no longer from the begin to the surrender of a game.

If you are having hassle napping, don't strain approximately it and attempt now not to stress your self as this can only make topics a whole lot worse.

The excellent approach for coping with sleeplessness isn't to assume however to act. So in area of with out end tossing and turning and clock-searching, get away from bed and do some difficulty like reading or searching TV.

Stay up till you experience tired sufficient to move back to mattress. The reason for getting up and studying or looking television is to direct your thoughts away from a few aspect it is that is maintaining you conscious.

Under no situations have to you begin wondering or fretting approximately the next day's exercise, if that's what's maintaining your mind energetic. Change your interest and your consciousness will exchange.

6.2.Four Focus

Focusing even as actively playing soccer may be less tough said than carried out as many will testify. It might be very vital, but, which you learn how to absolutely attention on the sport you are taking part in.

Don't permit your mind wander or end up distracted via something or someone else. If you do, you have got sincerely emerge as much less valuable on the arena.

One instance of strategies attention may be disrupted is if your train tells you to play out of position.

Even if you do not like the idea, you have to nevertheless placed any horrible thoughts from your head and without a doubt address the function you have been given.

Okay, so that you may not adore it, however it is although your task, and in times like this you certainly need to anticipate greater approximately the broader team strive than your very own dissatisfaction.

Other topics that could have an effect in your attention encompass the device you're using, the weather, the scenario of the pitch, non-public issues, screaming spectators, quite women inside the crowd, and so on and so forth.

Many beginner soccer gamers have a tendency no longer to rate the importance of attention an excessive amount of.

Indeed, they'll now not moreover be conscious that they outcomes lose popularity sooner or later of a sport. Yet all of the aforementioned gadgets are essential for playing high-quality soccer.

I might venture every person to play a game after a sleepless night time time, or with out right nutrients, and with a loss of attention, and be aware how they fare. Their universal overall performance, or lack or, would say all of it.

On the flip thing, playing football with all the aforementioned below manipulate, vitamins, relaxation, and cognizance, and the success degree might be in reality contrary to that of game enthusiasts who fall short in these areas.

6.Three Nutrition checklist

To assist you along with your football vitamins I in reality have composed a 12 thing soccer nutrients checklist. You may also additionally need to print this out and located it somewhere wherein it can not be prevented like on the fridge in any other case you mattress room door, as examples.

The 12 issue Soccer Nutrition checklist:

1. Aim to devour a balanced and awesome football weight loss program every day.

2.   Don't skip food. Energy intake is crucial in your soccer performance and should no longer be neglected.

three. Aim to contain your self in some shape physical interest every day, outdoor of exercise and video games.

4.   Ensure you sleep nicely as this may supply your body time to repair itself and convert meals into energy. Aim for among 7.Five to eight.Five hours a night time time. Don't sleep for extra than 8.Five hours or any an awful lot lots less than 7.Five hours if you are considered an "common sleeper".

5.   Fast food is not an green supply of power or nutrients. Furthermore, over-consuming fast and processed ingredients will reason you to benefit weight. The apparent quit end result of weight gain is probably that you become slower and much less responsive on the world. Get into the addiction of limiting your consumption of those types of food to as soon as every week or a whole lot much less.

6.   Healthy snacks include meals which encompass tremendous fats together with nuts, and easy fruits which provide you with an outstanding nutritional enhance.

7.   Calcium is crucial for sturdy bones. Low-fat calcium sources like milk, cheese, and yogurt are specific alternatives.

eight. Iron, which enables supply oxygen across the body, is a essential element for soccer fitness and fitness. Fill up on iron with the aid of manner of the usage of consuming beef and fowl.

nine.   A football weight loss plan also needs to contain zinc as this permits in boom and repair. It is critical for protective towards a few injuries too, and for healing gift injuries.

10.   Water must be your staple drink. Nothing quenches your thirst higher.

eleven.   When deciding on substances to snack on, commonly pick human beings with little to no fats, salt, and sugar content fabric.

12.   A choice of clean fruit is the healthiest and most dietary snack you can have.

Becoming the top notch player that you can likely be is all about determination, persistence, and incessant staying strength.

Follow the endorsed nutritional hints on this ebook and you have a exceptional basis on which to assemble your very very own soccer success story.

Chapter 7: Nutrition Pyramid Of Importance

Let us face it, you have were given were given first-class such loads of hours an afternoon, maximum of which may be spent unrelated to food. As with all matters, the more time you spend on some component, the extra know-how you will advantage, and the higher you turn into. However, much like how working towards passing and receiving is greater vital for a soccer player than training bicycle/overhead kicks, there are fantastic factors of vitamins as a way to provide larger consequences in a shorter time frame. Therefore, make some time rely via ensuring that you understand the Nutrition Pyramid of Importance.

To achieve the most out of your soccer vitamins, it's so important which you spend time at the more critical areas—like ingesting sufficient calories—and are not so concerned approximately subjects which deliver significantly less fee for your time and money. A close to buddy of mine, Michael Mroczka, may want to argue with me for years approximately the variety of energy I eat being greater critical than the high-quality of these energy even as striving to gain a purpose. Sadly, sometimes, I can be cussed and because of the fact I had look at hundreds of vitamins books, health magazines, fitness encyclopedias, and articles on eating wholesome, I believed that ingesting extra healthy substances may offer more benefit than looking the sort of energy I ate.

Then, 3 months earlier than my marriage ceremony, I employed a dietician to indicate me on my ingesting leading as a whole lot as my marriage, so I might be inside the outstanding form of my existence when I went to Jamaica for our honeymoon. Now, hold in mind that I have been eating extraordinarily healthy and workout a ton over the ten years preceding—now not to mention I had completed many at-domestic DVD workout packages, like P90X, Insanity, Body Beast, and so on. Sure enough, the dietician's vital cause for my entire 12-week meal plan was targeted round making sure I took within the proper kind of energy for my preferred frame and met the suggestions for the macronutrients of carbohydrates, fats, and protein. When hiring the dietician who knew my giant ancient past in vitamins, I knowledgeable him to tell me what I had to do, and no longer what I desired to pay attention him say. So, he stayed consistent approximately how vital the strength and macronutrition have been.

I had paid him lots to manual me, so I became dedicated to following his recommendation, irrespective of how a good deal I notion the great of the meals, taking nutritional dietary supplements, and meal timing end up greater important. Sure enough, on the stop of the 12-week length, I seemed the exceptional and maximum described I clearly have ever seemed in my lifestyles. From that aspect on, I discovered out I became incorrect and that the Nutrition Pyramid of Importance have grow to be key in figuring out how I spent my time.

For soccer game enthusiasts, understanding the Nutrition Pyramid of Importance will come up with an advantage over gamers who do no longer care approximately nutrition, and players who care about vitamins however popularity too much on taking lots of dietary supplements and consuming 8 times an afternoon.

Let us now speak every area of the Nutrition Pyramid of Importance and the way they will make a extensive impact. This is the longest financial disaster inside the e-book because it will provide an reason for the severa components of meals to make sure that you can resultseasily look at along thing the relaxation of the chapters.

Calories

When constructing a pyramid (or your frame), having a sturdy foundation will make it much less tough to assemble all other layers. At the bottom of the Nutrition Pyramid of Importance are power. A calorie is how we diploma the quantity of strength there may be in meals. Like how producing our international's energy from coal impacts the environment in a notable way than strength from wind, solar, or water, the energy from carbohydrates differs from protein or fat, and a calorie from a sweet bar is unique even as in comparison to a calorie from organic brown rice. Here are the advocated guidelines for the huge sort of energy to consume every day:

Now, you will be questioning that counting your energy can take some of time. Yes, it could. I from time to time spent hours a day getting geared up/measuring meals in the course of my 12-week meal plan previous to getting married. This is in reality too time consuming for max football game enthusiasts however statistics a way to look at a vitamins label (blanketed in a later financial disaster), and the manner to estimate the form of power and protein that you have eaten in a day will display whether or no longer or no longer your eating behavior will help you carry out better or preserve you lower back from fulfillment.

Macronutrients

Macronutrients are the carbs, fats, proteins, fibers, and fluids needed to feature. Macronutrients are favored in massive portions from food. Which ones you eat and even as you consume them can be the difference from having a six-percent and lean body or a mean body which goes neglected.

Carbs (carbohydrates) are broken down through using the frame to provide power from sugars, starches, and cellulose. For carbs, it's miles proper to classify them into classes: speedy-digesting and sluggish-digesting. Fast-digesting carbs are the such things as white bread, white rice, and white pasta which your body can speedy trade into blood sugar (glycogen), which reasons a pointy spike to your body's blood sugar. This can be genuine on the equal time as you are approximately to carry out in a football pastime or at the identical time as consuming a positioned up-undertaking protein shake. However, it is able to be terrible in your frame at different elements of the day whilst you do now not want prolonged power/sugar levels and do no longer want to enjoy a "crash" of strength. Foods like oatmeal, whole wheat pasta, sweet potatoes, brown rice, and entire grain bread are an entire lot slower digesting and reason sustained levels of power at the same time as no longer having spikes and dips in strength.

Fats (lipids) are in particular essential to offer your frame power, guide cellular boom, shield your organs, hold your body warmness, soak up fat-soluble nutrients, and bring essential hormones. Fats are to be had in 4 important types: 1) Monounsaturated 2) Polyunsaturated 3) Saturated four) Trans. Both monounsaturated and polyunsaturated fats are healthy. Fats from nuts, seeds, olives, algae, and fatty fish will provide the unsaturated fat desired. These varieties of fats are liquid at room temperature.

Saturated fat are solid at room temperature and can be placed in palm and coconut oils, cheese, butter, and pork. Currently, the fitness community is torn on whether or now not the ones are wholesome fat or not. Personally, it is hard to mention that a coconut is horrific for you. There are such pretty some benefits of coconut oil that I should write a whole book on them. Feel free to do more studies at the venture, however I in truth accept as proper with primarily based on severa research that high-quality natural cheeses, butter, and pink meats moderately will result in a extra healthful manner of life for a soccer participant than maintaining off them actually.

Also, there are trans-fat. There are a few clearly taking region trans-unsaturated fatty acids in meat and milk fat. However, the genuine "villain" of fat is trans-fat, this is chemically created in a production facility thru hydrogenating oils. This way that meals companies turn liquid oils into solids to increase the shelf life and taste of the substances which incorporate them. There is currently a large fashion within the health business corporation to avoid the ones fat because of the fact they'll be linked to coronary coronary heart disease. The trick to seeing if there is trans-fat in a packaged ideal is to check the additives listing for any in aspect or genuinely hydrogenated oils and live as a long way a long way from them as you could.

Like carbohydrates, protein can be seemed with the beneficial aid of the way speedy it digests. First, protein is made from many amino acids, which help useful useful resource in everyday cellular feature, muscle boom, enzyme creation, hormone production, and they may be used for power. Whey protein—which comes from milk—is one of the fastest-digesting proteins. It may be sold separately from milk, too. Casein protein— which also comes from milk—is one of the slowest-digesting proteins. The protein from fish/shellfish is faster digesting than the protein from red meat, while chook/turkey falls in among. Think of protein as your muscle's constructing blocks.

Lastly, the very last macronutrient we are capable of cowl is fiber. Technically, fiber is a carbohydrate. However, it's far a carb which the body can't digest. Fiber is essential for regulating digestion, regular bowel moves, enables hold you feeling fuller for longer, improves your levels of cholesterol, regulates blood sugar levels, and prevents illnesses like diabetes and coronary coronary heart sickness. Fiber is often classified in considered considered certainly one of approaches: 1) Soluble 2) Insoluble. Soluble fiber dissolves in water and in gastrointestinal fluids at the same time as it enters your frame's belly and intestines. It modifications proper into a gel-like substance that micro organism in your frame digests, releasing gases and a few electricity. Insoluble fiber does not dissolve in water or for your body and remains unchanged because it movements via you earlier than being pooped out. Because it isn't digested the least bit, insoluble fiber is not a deliver of energy your frame can use for power. Think of insoluble fiber as a cleanser which travels thru your body scrubbing down the walls and leaving the whole lot a touch bit extra healthy. Soluble fiber is in oat bran, barley, nuts, seeds, beans, lentils, peas, and some culmination and veggies. Insoluble fiber is in wheat bran, veggies, entire grains, and lots of others.

If the explanations of every of these macronutrients regarded excessive, don't worry. There is a fair much less hard manner to consider what is right to eat and what isn't always: If it became made in a manufacturing unit, then it might be now not true for you. In popular, end result, greens, natural grains, sustainably raised meats, nuts, seeds, beans, and fish are right for you. They may be located in nature. Processed food, packaged gadgets, and beverages are made by using the usage of human beings in a manufacturing facility and commonly are not true for you.

Micronutrients

A micronutrient is an element or substance this is required in trace quantities for normal increase and improvement. Micronutrients can be damaged down into the following key areas: nutrients, minerals, antioxidants, and phytonutrients. Vitamins and minerals are essential for appropriate health. Antioxidants, anti-inflammatories, and phytonutrients are not important, however they are beneficial for recovery, ailment prevention, and pain cut charge.

Consuming enough nutrients from meals and supplements is vital due to the truth the frame can't produce enough on its own. There are thirteen vital nutrients, and they will be all water-soluble or fat-soluble. Fat-soluble vitamins can dissolve in fats and oils. They are absorbed along side fats inside the weight-reduction plan and can be stored inside the frame's fat shops, which makes them the simpler of the two for the frame to preserve. Vitamins A, D, E, and K are fats-soluble. Water-soluble nutrients are carried all through the body but aren't stored in the frame, so that they've to be taken in every day. Vitamins B and C are water-soluble.

Minerals are important in your body to live wholesome. Your body makes use of minerals to assemble your bones, to have interaction your muscle groups, create enzymes, produce hormones, alter your blood, enhance metabolism, and hold your stressful machine. There are kinds of minerals: 1) Macrominerals 2) Trace Minerals. They encompass calcium, phosphorus, magnesium, sodium, potassium, chloride, and sulfur. You only need small quantities of trace minerals. They embody iron, manganese, copper, iodine, zinc, cobalt, fluoride, and selenium. Your body dreams large portions of macrominerals than hint minerals.

Antioxidants are virtually "anti" oxidants. Oxidants are produced interior your frame and outside within the surroundings, and they will react with specific factors for your body, collectively with protein, DNA, and fats. The oxidants will damage your frame and purpose illnesses like most cancers, and contamination like arthritis. Therefore, antioxidants prevent harm from the oxidants. Antioxidants slow or prevent harm to cells because of unfastened radicals, which is probably volatile molecules in your body.

As an instance, if grill marks are burned into your chicken breast due to the reality you cooked it on the grill, the burned marks are oxidants to your body. However, in case you eat some broccoli and blueberries with the chicken breast, then the antioxidants from the broccoli and blueberries ought to assist combat the oxidants from the blistered elements of the grilled chicken.

Phytonutrients are what deliver end result and vegetables their shade. Below, the particular forms of phytonutrients are listed. However, remembering their names is not critical. The key to remembering phytonutrients is understanding the five sunglasses and ensuring you're consuming each of the colours:

Red: Protects your DNA whilst preventing maximum cancers and coronary coronary heart sickness.

Foods: Apples, pomegranates, grapefruits, cherries, tomatoes, radishes, watermelons, raspberries, strawberries, and so forth.

Blue/Purple: Good for coronary coronary heart, thoughts, bones, and arteries. Fights most cancers and promotes wholesome growing old.

Foods: Plums, crimson cabbage, beets, eggplants, purple grapes, blueberries, blackberries, and so forth.

Green: Support eye health, arteries, lungs, and liver feature. Helps to heal wounds and gum fitness.

Foods: Broccoli, kale, spinach, collard veggies, kiwis, avocados, honeydews, lettuce, celery, and so on.

White: Supports bone fitness, circulatory device, and arteries. Helps fight heart illness and most cancers.

Foods: Onions, mushrooms, pears, garlic, cauliflower, parsnips, and lots of others.

Yellow/Orange: Good for eye health, immune feature, and healthful development.

Foods: Pineapples, peaches, papayas, bananas, lemons, carrots, pumpkins, sweet potatoes, nectarines, and so on.

According to WebMD.Com, 4 out of five people do not consume sufficient end result and greens. Although greens offer few proteins, fats, or carbs (other than fiber), they're vital for their fiber, vitamins, minerals, antioxidants, and phytonutrients.

Meal Timing/Frequency

Meal timing is making plans meals and snacks for particular instances at a few degree in the day (e.G., after a exercising) to govern hunger, resource recuperation, gasoline performance, enhance sleep, and build muscle.

Meal frequency is how regularly you eat. For example, the common individual eats 3 instances in step with day with one snack. However, a soccer participant might also moreover moreover discover it higher for their wishes to consume 5 times in step with day and characteristic a publish-exercising shake after training.

When meal timing, the maximum crucial element to recollect is whether or not you're ingesting a put up-workout shake in case you are schooling intensely, and to make sure which you are consuming at the least 3 food consistent with day that consist of the large variety of strength you need to gain your ideal body.

Chapter 8: Making A Routine

We are what we again and again do. Excellence, therefore, isn't an act, but a addiction."

Aristotle

Routines/habits are so essential for finding achievement results easily and undertaking your goals. When you start a few details new, there may be frequently pleasure, anxiety, and fear. You are harassed about reading some element new and must use severa intellectual power to start and keep the way to discover approximately that new scenario. Excitingly, this "10-foot hurdle" that most people region in their minds typically first-rate looks as if a 6-inch pace bump after you've got got lengthy gone over it. Starting, committing, and learning the things you do no longer understand is often the most difficult a part of starting, but as soon as you've got were given the difficult stuff out of the way, it turns into a bargain much less complex from there.

However, the trouble maximum human's face is they spend a lot time and strength the primary few activities doing something which they suppose every single time can be like that and require masses of effort. The following photo suggests how maximum human beings view subjects they recognize they need to be doing, like ingesting wholesome and exercise.

They give up without figuring out they'll be close to attending to the point in which it's far going to be smooth to hold. Therefore, growing a routine takes a large quantity of try to devour healthy, workout, read, achieve enough sleep, and plenty of others. However, it turns into so smooth to preserve as quickly as you have created a system (i.E., ordinary/way/dependancy). Instead, have a look at the following photo for what it genuinely takes to keep a everyday going.

Notice inside the photograph it takes a number of physical attempt and intellectual strength up the the front to research the entirety and create the dependancy, but it most effective takes a piece of protection to preserve the dependancy going. So, how prolonged does it take to make a ordinary stick? Phillippa Lally, a fitness psychology researcher at University College London, posted a have a look at within the European Journal of Social Psychology on how long it takes to shape a dependancy. The have a look at examined the behavior of individuals over a 12-week period. Each character decided on one new addiction for the 12 weeks and advised every day on whether or not or no longer they did the behavior and the manner automated the addiction changed into.

Because the individuals need to pick out out out their very own behavior, some were more difficult than others. At the give up of the 12 weeks, the researchers analyzed the information to determine how long it took anybody to head from beginning a contemporary behavior to automatically doing it. On commonplace, it sixty six days for the new addiction to paste. It took less time for less difficult obligations and longer for more tough exercises. Also, how prolonged it took severa depending on the character and the activities. Therefore, 66 days or honestly over months is a splendid aim to installation the habitual of creating equipped meals and ingesting wholesome. The researchers also determined that it did now not count if the human beings tousled now and then. Building higher behavior isn't an all-or-now not something system when putting in the recurring.

Given this ebook is prepared nutrients for the soccer participant, permit us to speak about the most crucial regular in vitamins—what to devour and what form of of it. The above photo of "MyPlate" indicates the breakout of the way the U.S. Department of Agriculture recommends we detail our food. Remember that as a soccer player, your nutritional desires are one-of-a-type in comparison to the general population given that you workout hundreds extra. More workout approach you want more gas to perform well and need to apprehend whilst to consume every sort of meals to assist with recuperation with out decreasing your electricity.

Therefore, have a observe the subsequent picture for a better recommendation for a football player. Feel unfastened to exchange it based totally for your ideals and what works exceptional to your body.

Now, preserve in mind that the serving period for an eight-year-vintage lady could be considered one of a kind than a 15-twelve months-vintage boy, however fruits and greens ought to be a staple of each meal plan. Notice that the photo is a pyramid, rather than a plate. A plate indicates which you want to consume the same five food groups in every meal, even as the pyramid is not as restrictive and permits you to better plan food round a education session or undertaking with a serving duration equal to at least one cup. Also, the pyramid offers a few more property you need to devour, together with water as the muse to ensure that your frame will remain hydrated. You can be the healthiest eater for your organization, but in case you are dehydrated in advance than the begin of a enterprise, then properly success outperforming a person who can also moreover moreover have eaten worse materials but is nicely-hydrated!

Here are examples of things to devour from every "meals enterprise":

Healthy Fats – Coconut Oil, Extra-Virgin Olive Oil, & Avocado Oil

Dairy – Organic Milk, Greek Yogurt, & Minimally-Processed Cheese

Meats/Proteins – Beef, Poultry, Fish, Eggs, Beans, Nuts, & Seeds

Grains – Whole Grain Breads, Rice, Potatoes, Pasta, Organic Corn, & Steel-Cut Oatmeal

Fruits – Melons, Berries, Apples, Pears, Bananas, Peaches, Grapes, & Oranges

Vegetables – Lettuce, Carrots, Onions, Celery, Kale, Cabbage, Broccoli, Cauliflower, & Celery

Water – Not sports drinks, no longer flavored water drinks, and no longer soda pop.

Because this bankruptcy is all about developing routines, permit us to speak severa strategies to make it less difficult to devour wholesome:

1. Cook in bulk (meal prep). By cooking in bulk, you could make it less complicated to supply food with you and generally have a few element healthful prepared. Having such severa unique obligations (e.G., college, work, chores, family, buddies, and lots of others.) way that having meals already made will make the recurring of eating healthy even much less tough.

2. Keep smooth-to-draw close end result and veggies available. Having give up result and greens that take minimum or no time to put together will make eating healthful greater exciting. Having to put together a few factor rather than grabbing a bag of chips makes it much more likely which you grab the chips. However, deciding on among a bag of chips

and an apple will boom your probabilities of making a greater nutritious choice because of the truth you do not need prepare an apple, orange, container of raisins, carrots, or celery. For instance, as soon as I am in a hurry, I can effects clutch a banana, some pieces of cabbage, a slice of herbal complete-grain bread, and a handful of nuts. These clean-to-capture gadgets do now not want to be prepared; I without a doubt have to pick out them up and take them with me.

3. Remove risky food from the house. Getting horrible food out of your home will make it even a lot less complex to devour healthful due to the reality you can now not want to apply any strength of thoughts to choose out out among healthy and perilous components if dangerous ingredients are not an opportunity, a concept called "preference shape." If you're the individual that stores in your own family, then make certain you do now not visit the grocery keep hungry. If you aren't the person who shops for your own family, then it'll in all likelihood be a bit

greater hard to get the meals that you want. The best issue to do right right here is to talk to the person that does the grocery buying to satisfaction buy the extra wholesome and clean-to-seize alternatives you need. However, you can have a figure who does no longer need to buy greater wholesome substances. Sadly, I had this, and it limited my food alternatives for a while in the residence earlier than my mom commenced purchasing for substances that I may also eat. You owe it to yourself, your health, and your performance on the football discipline to have the communique with the individual that buys the food.

four. Establish a regular for what your "everyday" meal need to seem like. Knowing what a "ordinary" meal seems like makes it less tough to realise what need to be in your plate. A remarkable meal includes one vegetable, one meat/protein, one fruit, and one grain (i.E., carb). Remember this! Honestly, ninety five% of my food comply with this easy-to-bear in mind pattern, which takes away the hard artwork of selecting what to consume. If that your food should have 4 key food corporations, then it's far a great deal much less difficult to put together/clutch them. This addiction will help you grow to be hundreds healthier and perform better on the soccer location. For instance, as I am writing this chapter, I grabbed a stalk of celery (i.E., vegetable), walnuts (i.E., protein), raisins (i.E., fruit), and a sweet potato (i.E., grain/carb) to gas the 2 hours of futsal (i.E., 5v5 indoor football) which I play on Fridays.

In precis, information how prolonged it takes to form a routine, which behavior will reason a healthful way of life, and which suggestions will benefit you can make ingesting extra healthy pretty smooth to do. Remember that maximum conduct take a considerable amount of strength and try and set up however as speedy as created, they'll be typically with out issues maintained. Therefore, continuously do something with the cause of creating it a dependancy. Creating conduct like ingesting wholesome, exercise regularly, getting sufficient sleep, and studying/listening to proper books will ultimately turn you into the character you want to be.

Chapter 9: Why Dieting Is Bad

Your relationship with food and the way you view it makes a massive distinction on the way you sense and the manner you appearance. So many humans have "Yo-Yo" diets wherein they'll start a weight loss program for some weeks, devour some junk-crammed meals, say they want to be higher, after which preserve consuming extra meals void of nutrients to cowl their bad emotions approximately falling off their food plan. This maintains for some months and then they get decrease returned on some different diet and change once more. Honestly, surely seeking to give an reason behind that is onerous and the Yo-Yo weight-reduction plan does now not artwork. It is really too tough to move for prolonged durations of time with out the meals you want and then to binge consume them whilst you slip up.

Instead, what I virtually have determined works exceptional is not considering it as a "weight loss program." Rather, think about it as a manner of lifestyles—the way in which you'll stay. Because the phrase "healthy eating plan" has such a lot of awful emotions and feelings round it for most humans, you will be extra a success with the aid of no longer viewing your meal plan as a weight loss plan. The hassle with diets is they forestall. Remember the dietician I employed to create a "food plan" for me for the 12 weeks number one as heaps as my marriage ceremony? Well, he helped me lose 14 pounds. Guess what took place as quickly as I went off my weight loss program. I obtained 14 kilos in 14 days. I had limited what I ate for what appeared like forever that I began consuming an excessive amount of as soon as I modified into off the food regimen. I swung within the extraordinary course due to the fact I turned into not at the diet regime.

Therefore, it is an entire lot much less hard to have some carrying sports and rules in vicinity which you comply with 90 5% of the time. People regularly will say "I dislike having suggestions due to the fact it is so constricting." If you view it this manner, you then definately actually are right. However, having a few rules similar to the order you devour your meals, ensuring you devour remarkable food 90 5% of the time, how masses you workout, and many others. Clearly loose you up for one-of-a-kind subjects. As noted within the habitual bankruptcy, as soon as you've got were given the habitual and addiction in location, it is so clean to hold. The regulations create freedom due to the truth you do no longer need to spend time and strength deciding on what you have to and have to not consume. Rules make it much less complicated to win. These guidelines are higher called a "life-style." Something to do for the relaxation of your existence.

You are one exchange away within the way you view food and exercise from being able to be very healthful. Do I although eat burgers, do I consume cakes, do I even have cookies near Christmas? The answer is positive to every this type of questions. I virtually have truely virtually taken the time to parent out my regulations which allow me to experience lifestyles and permit me to feel good about my ability to perform on the soccer concern and look appropriate doing it.

After years and years of appearing plastic surgical treatment operations, Dr. Maxwell Maltz exhibits in his excellent-selling e-book, Psycho-Cybernetics, that a person commonly aligns with their self-picture. This is specifically essential. People who be given as genuine with they may be obese can make the alternatives of an in-shape individual over the following couple of weeks, but they commonly "snap lower back" to their view of themselves. Therefore, inside the event that they view themselves as someone who will typically be obese, then they make the same horrible ingesting selections and lack of exercising that they continually have.

Make certain that you take a minute and ask yourself what your perspectives are related to food, the way you experience, the way you appearance, and in case you weigh the right quantity or too much. Now, it isn't to say that it's far best "to your head." Saying this may be a piece insulting. Instead, it's miles based on idea styles that, when modified, will deliver the outcomes you need. As an instance, I mentally view myself as someone who will usually be healthful and healthy. I changed my self-photo earlier than I have been given fit to help gain the body that I preferred.

To make it simpler to align with a "healthy" self-photo, a trick is to recognition on the ingredients you like. Of all the vegetables to be had, my 3 favorites are carrots, lettuce, and sautéed onions. I love cease stop result, meats, and maximum grains/carbs. So, what did I do to gather success? I installation my manner of life and meal plan focusing at the subjects I enjoy. Will you ever see me consuming an artichoke? Nope. Artichokes disgust me and make my flavor buds harm just thinking about it. Being capable of find out healthy food you need will make it winnable to obtain a better self-photo.

In conclusion, this bankruptcy is all about difficult the manner you view yourself-picture and your manner of life. If you view it as "I need to be on a diet," then you may in all likelihood fail. Instead, in case you view your meals alternatives as locating what you enjoy and growing a way of life, then you will be for your way to achievement. Having the self-photo of a healthful and physical wholesome man or woman is a great difficulty. Finally, ingesting healthy does not need to be difficult; at the opposite, even as you consume healthier, all the components you consume taste better. Imagine eating a slice of watermelon, or each unique fruit you enjoy. It tastes especially proper, right? Now, do not forget eating a slice of watermelon after consuming candy bars. It will not taste so properly due to the fact your taste buds have end up used to the sugar rush from terrible candies. Therefore, in case you devour extra healthful elements, then while you eat fruit, it will flavor like candy.

Chapter 10: Pre-Game And In-Game Nutrition

Your pre-game meal(s) can set you up for achievement or can motive you to fail. A man or woman consuming a meal comprising steak, cottage cheese, entire milk, cheese, and cashews might also have unique energy ranges than the person that eats carrots, watermelon, fish, and rice in advance than a sport. Therefore, allow us to damage down the meals to include within the hours fundamental as an awful lot as a recreation to ensure you have got had been given a ton of energy even as you want it most.

What to Eat the Morning of a Game

Upon awakening, your frame has used up most of its excess blood sugar stores (glycogen) sooner or later of the night time time, so eat meals which might be better in carbohydrates. Examples are give up result, greens, and healthful grains along with quinoa, brown rice, sweet potatoes, metal-lessen oatmeal, and natural complete grain bread.

These carbohydrates are beneficial to top off your body's blood-sugar stores and give you the electricity that will help you function because it have to be until your next meal. There is a common false impression in the athletic global that you are supposed to "carb up" the night time earlier than a activity. For example, many corporations should have a pasta dinner the night time time before a enterprise, thinking this can assist them benefit enough carbs to be completely fueled for the game tomorrow. It is actual that consuming some carbohydrates is a superb detail in advance than a schooling consultation, however you do now not need to devour three bowls of pasta the night time earlier than a venture. Eating too many carbs the night time time earlier than a recreation will growth the chances that they will be saved in the frame as fat.

Also, a awesome recommendation for the morning of a endeavor is to a eat a few protein. However, keep away from dairy merchandise! Furthermore, there are better alternatives than nuts, seeds, and beans previous to your activity. Instead, eat a few eggs or faster digesting property of protein like chicken, turkey, or fish. Personally, scrambled eggs paintings quality for me because of the reality I can put together them with onions (a vegetable) and make severa servings right now. This is extraordinary to have as a wholesome grab-and-cross desire within the morning on the identical time as you are regularly moved rapid and rushed to get out the door.

What to Eat as your Last Meal Before Your Game Starts

It is useful a good way to consume carbs within the path of endeavor time, however this is predicated upon on how well your frame digests food and the manner empty or complete you opt to be whilst gambling soccer. Often, one to a few hours before the begin of the sport is an remarkable time to absorb extra carbohydrates inside the form of faster-digesting vegetables, which incorporates carrots; culmination together with apples, bananas, or watermelon, further to carbs inclusive of quinoa, sweet potatoes, or brown rice. Furthermore, eat turkey, fish, or grilled bird to ensure you've got were given some protein too and to preserve you fuller for longer. One final element to recollect is if there may be ever a time to characteristic salt for your meal, preceding to a recreation would be the fine time to do it. Your muscle businesses want salts which contain minerals like sodium, potassium, and magnesium to agreement and art work effectively. So, in advance than those long video video video games or video games in mainly heat temperatures, ingesting a bit of salt will assist your muscle agencies function nicely and assist you preserve more water to make certain you stay hydrated.

Pre-Game Supplement

Many football players do no longer drink a pre-exercising/pre-sport supplement. However, that is frequently to the detriment of the player due to the reality it could increase their overall performance thru 10-15% and is regularly used by special gamers on the arena. Many game enthusiasts use lesser versions of pre-exercising blends along with carbonated soda pop or energy liquids. The problem with these is all the filler components, synthetic flavors, and artificial preservatives which are not suitable to your health. You will study greater about which pre-workout supplement to take inside the subsequent economic ruin, however apprehend that it is encouraged, and I take one too.

In-Game Nutrition

In 90 5% of practices/video video games, you do no longer want in-exercise nutrition. Drinking a sports activities activities drink on an incredibly warm day if you have a endeavor that lasts more than an hour is suitable but for maximum games, you already have enough vitamins in your frame if you ate nicely earlier than the sport. Your body is constructed from 70% water, so drink plenty of it!

As you can see, there are several topics to make sure you have power on undertaking day. Also, this identical expertise may be used at the same time as you try out for a set too. If you have got were given were given a tryout springing up, recollect grabbing the Understand Soccer collection ebook, Soccer Tryouts, to analyze all the subjects to help you make the organization and believe from the begin with out being worrying. For pre-recreation nutrients, keep in mind that faster digesting materials like bird and fish, greens, forestall end result, and grains/carbs are your amazing bets previous to undertaking time to make sure the entirety in your machine is supporting you perform at your pinnacle. Consider a pre-exercise supplement to apply quality earlier than video video video games to provide you a boost and don't worry about in-undertaking nutrients other than water.

YouTube: If you would really like to observe a video on what to eat earlier than football, then hold in thoughts watching the Understand Soccer YouTube video: What to Eat Before a Soccer Game.

Chapter 11: Supplements

Pre-Workout/Game

Ever enjoy along with you do not have enough strength to perform properly on the sphere? Well, pre-workout dietary supplements can give you the physical decorate and mental soar begin which you need. The preference on whether or no longer or not to take a pre-exercise supplement preceding to a game will range from individual to person. Personally, I will take a incredible pre-exercise complement to provide me more power in the course of crucial video video games. It is essential to have sufficient energy to show off your skills and abilties. However, for the purpose that I am no longer an authorized clinical physician, please are searching for advice out of your doctor earlier than taking a pre-exercise supplement.

Also, keep in thoughts that at the least 80% of the pre-workout dietary supplements available on the market are not advocated. They are full of synthetic shades, flavors, sweeteners, and typically have quite some filler additives, which make it appear to be you are becoming extra in your coins. However, you're awesome getting a group of chemical materials, at the way to purpose lengthy-term issues.

Instead, skip for a pre-exercising complement with only a few excessive-powered additives—the most important being caffeine. Caffeine is a vital worried device stimulant, which offers you power and highbrow cognizance. Caffeine takes impact approximately forty five mins while you eat it. While caffeine is beneficial to your conventional performance on the sphere, the results of caffeinated beverages (e.G., tea, espresso, pre-exercise dietary supplements, energy beverages, or carbonated soda pop) lasts for 4-6 hours, so keep away from consuming caffeine in the 6 hours prior to bedtime to decrease its effect on your rest.

One of my endorsed pre-workout nutritional supplements is Pure Pump. Pure Pump has the depended on factors you need in a pre-exercising complement with none of the fluff. This product is for every men and women. I am no longer backed with the useful resource of this company; I simply in reality like this product due to the fact they do not add unnecessary materials. Personally, I eat the unflavored version, however I advocate the flavored model due to the fact the unflavored model tastes a piece metal. One scoop works well for youngsters, and two scoops is the endorsed serving length for an individual.

When you're taking any kind of pre-workout supplement, make certain to drink at the least eight oz.. Of water with it.

Post-Workout/Game

Ever surprise what could assist you fine get higher after a education session, exercising, or exercise in that 30-minute window on the same time as your body virtually wishes vitamins to broaden stronger? Well, meals that are proper to consume after a workout are meals high in carbohydrates and speedy-digesting protein. An example of a food that is simple to advantage is herbal milk. Though the proof shows converting views on lactose, having a few natural milk or a whey protein shake with non-GMO dextrose is beneficial after a enterprise. You want to take in enough carbohydrates to spike up your blood sugar after a exercising, recreation, or workout in order that your frame uses the protein that you'll absorb.

In terms of a supplement to apply, whey protein isolate is recommended due to the reality it's far one of the most bio-available and fastest digesting proteins. (Whey protein pay interest is a whole lot much less luxurious, but it has masses of fat and lactose that may purpose stinky flatulence. Whey protein hydrolysate is the exceptional, however it is nearly double the charge of whey protein isolate. Whey protein hydrolysate does no longer offer even close to two times the benefits of whey protein isolate and ought to notable be considered if fee does not be counted number to you.) If you drink milk, it has milk protein, it's 20% whey protein and 80% casein protein. It is vital that if you have greater physical sports later inside the day, take in sufficient carbohydrates like dextrose, bread, rice, potatoes, pasta, and oatmeal to refill your glycogen. It is critical to decrease the amount of fats and fiber which you absorb at a few diploma in the put up-exercising 30-minute window because fiber and fats are slower digesting. They gradual the absorption of vitamins, minerals, and nutrients. Avoid very dense meals like spinach or peanut butter except there can be in reality no longer something else that you may eat. Something healthful is higher than nothing.

The distinct recommended positioned up-workout complement is creatine monohydrate. More than a thousand studies have tested that creatine is a top complement for exercise overall performance. Creatine is a mixture of three critical amino acids: glycine, arginine, and methionine. Consuming creatine will boom your stores of phosphocreatine, that could be a shape of stored energy in the cells that allows your frame produce more immoderate-strength ATP. ATP is called the frame's "electricity forex." When you've got were given got greater ATP, you carry out higher at some stage in football. Creatine additionally allows severa strategies that boom muscle tissues and electricity and lift recuperation. If you worry approximately taking some element as distant places sounding as creatine monohydrate, then recognize that there are one to two grams of creatine in a pound of beef, and ranging portions in specific red meats, dairy, chicken, and fish.

If you need to determine out which supplement you're interested by, take a look at out labdoor.Com! They go through maximum nutritional dietary supplements and do the research on which ones are wholesome and which ones are not, so you must have more time for soccer.

General Health

To hold fitness and fitness, the very last topics to keep in mind are a multivitamin, and a fish-oil complement. Think of a multivitamin as "insurance." By following the suggestions on this ebook and eating healthy food (e.G., fruits, vegetables, meat, grains, and dairy), you will gather the nutrients and minerals you want. However, simply in case there may be a fantastic food which you aren't eating with dietary fee that is not positioned in different components, a multivitamin can help make up for what your meal plan lacks.

Lastly, a fish oil supplement is ideal too. Fish oil has been shown to:

1.Support coronary heart fitness.

2.Treat mental problems.

3.Aid in weight reduction

4.Support eye health.

5.Reduce contamination.

6.Support healthful pores and skin.

7.Reduce liver fats.

8.Reduce despair.

nine.Reduce attention deficit problems.

10.Improve bronchial bronchial asthma.

eleven.Help bone fitness.

In summary, a pre-exercise supplement will growth your electricity for crucial video video video games and tryouts. Post-exercise nutritional dietary supplements like whey protein isolate and creatine boom energy and muscle building at the same time as shortening the time to get higher. Finally, a multivitamin acts as a fantastic way to no longer worry approximately missing any key vitamins for your meal plan at the equal time as fish oil helps with such plenty of subjects that it's miles an crucial part of regular health and properly being.

Chapter 12: Post-Game Nutrition

After your exercise is completed, and you took a put up-pastime supplement, your body is primed to use the nutrients that you eat to restore it and bring together your muscle companies. Soccer game enthusiasts have exercise and/or video games numerous times regular with week, so it's miles right to absorb nutrients so one can help your muscle tissues get higher quicker and ensure which you are not fatigued in advance than the begin of your subsequent pastime.

Consume a meal much like the one you ate hours earlier than the sport started. Include one meat, one fruit, one vegetable, and one carb/grain to assist your frame recover from the intense recreation. If you do no longer revel in that you worked hard sufficient in the game to eat all this meals, then do not forget eliminating the carb/grain. If you consume nicely after your pastime, then you may carry out higher, faster, and greater effectively subsequent time.

Before mattress, you want a slower digesting meal, so devour meals excessive in fiber, excessive in fat, and immoderate in protein. Some subjects to don't forget eating are nuts, seeds, meat, remarkable nut butters (almond, cashew, and to a lesser quantity, peanut butter). Also, greens are constantly amazing to devour. Personally, I devour five servings of greens a day because of the fact they assist hold you whole for longer. Vegetables embody vitamins, minerals, antioxidants, and phytonutrients which help you get better quicker, keep you feeling higher, and help to maintain everyday blood sugar tiers so your energy tiers do no longer spike and crash. Additionally, in case you choose out to devour dairy merchandise and aren't lactose illiberal, then earlier than bed is one of the fine instances to eat them.

Cheese, Greek yogurt, whole milk (ideally organic), and cottage cheese will do a amazing system of providing muscle-repairing nutrients for your body for optimum of the night time time time. Dairy's milk protein is crafted from 20% whey protein, and eighty% casein protein. Casein protein takes up to seven hours to digest, which makes it a exceptional pre-bedtime protein to assist your body get better and gain energy. Avoid meals with an entire lot of carbohydrates (i.E., carbs) right in advance than bedtime because of the reality the carbohydrates can spike your blood-sugar, that could make it more difficult to go to sleep and growth the possibilities that the meals you truely ate may be saved as fats, in preference to used as fuel.

Example Meal Plan for a three p.M. Game

Breakfast (8 AM):

three eggs (protein & fats)

½ sautéed onion (vegetable)

½ cup of oatmeal (carb)

1 orange (non-obligatory fruit/carb)

Lunch (midday):

eight oz of grilled chicken breast (protein)

1 cup of carrots (vegetable)

1 apple (fruit/carb)

1-2 slices of natural bread (carb)

Snack (as needed):

1 banana (fruit/carb)

2 organic rice cakes (carb)

Pre-Workout (half-hour earlier than pastime time):

1-2 scoops of pre-exercise (more power)

1-2 cups of water (muscle healing and hydration)

Game (3 PM)

Post-Workout (5 PM):

1 scoop of whey protein isolate (muscle healing and growth)

1-2 cups of milk or water (muscle restoration and growth)

5 grams of creatine (muscle recuperation and increase)

Dinner (6 PM):

8 oz.. Of turkey, red meat, chicken, or fish (protein & fats)

1 cup of broccoli (vegetable)

1 cup of blueberries (fruit/carb)

1 sweet potato (carb)

30 Minutes Before Bed (10 PM):

½ cup of nuts (protein & fats)

4 oz. Of herbal cheese (protein & fat)

1-2 cups of leafy greens (vegetable)

1 cup of Greek yogurt or cottage cheese (protein & fats)

Example Meal Plan for a Daylong Tournament with 3 Games

Breakfast (5:30 AM):

3 eggs (protein)

½ sautéed onion (vegetable)

½ cup of oatmeal (carb)

1 orange (fruit/carb)

Pre-Game (30 minutes earlier than undertaking time):

1 scoop of pre-workout (extra power)

Game (7 AM)

Snack (8:45 AM):

1 banana (fruit – carb)

2 herbal rice cakes (carb)

Pre-Game (half of-hour earlier than undertaking time):

½ scoop of pre-exercise (more power)

1 cup of water (muscle recovery and hydration)

Game (eleven AM)

Lunch (1:00 PM):

eight oz of grilled fowl breast (protein)

1 cup of carrots (vegetable)

1 apple (fruit/carb)

1-2 slices of natural bread (carb)

Pre-Game (30 minutes in advance than sport time):

½ scoop of pre-exercising (extra electricity)

1 cup of water (muscle recovery and hydration)

Game (3 PM)

Post-Game Shake (5 PM):

1 scoop of whey protein isolate (muscle healing and boom)

2 cups of milk or water (muscle recovery and increase)

five grams of creatine (muscle restoration and boom)

Dinner (6 PM):

eight ounces of turkey, red meat, hen, or fish (protein & fat)

1 cup of broccoli (vegetable)

1 cup of blueberries (fruit/carb)

1-2 cups of whole wheat pasta (carb)

30 Minutes Before Bed (nine:30 PM):

½ cup of nuts (protein & fats)

four ozOf herbal cheese (protein & fat)

1-2 cups of leafy veggies (vegetable)

1 cup of Greek yogurt or cottage cheese (protein & fat)

Note: This is a high-quality meal plan for an person. If you're a little one or are analyzing this to help your little one, then reduce the element sizes more or lots less in half. Make substitutions wherein vital based on food alternatives. Each segment is classified (i.E., protein, vegetable, fruit, carb) to make it much less hard in case you need to alternate out something you or your infant does now not like. For example, use fruit interchangeably and vegetables too (i.E., eating watermelon in place of a banana is exquisite and so is ingesting celery in preference to broccoli.)

Chapter 13: Renaldo's And Mess's Meal Plans

For an effective meal plan, it's far often crucial to examine a number of the great gamers to find out what they are consuming and to apply it as a tenet for what you ought to eat. Specifically, in case you observed your desired celeb ingesting junk meals in advance than video games, you might be more likely to consider that eating healthily does not remember too much. However, in case you see the nice gamers having a nicely-balanced meal plan, then it is more likely that you can check their recommendation to enhance your exercise. Let us have a look at what Cristiano Ronaldo and Lionel Messi eat to stay on the pinnacle of their activity. For Cristiano Ronaldo, we will test what he eats over the path of an average day. For Lionel Messi, you could have a look at how he modifications up his meal plan depending how far away is his subsequent big in shape.

Cristiano Ronaldo's Daily Meal Plan

From huge research of Cristiano Ronaldo's consuming conduct, as verified in the pics on his Instagram account, he divides his every day food intake into 5 to six smaller meals to prevent susceptible point or starvation during the day and provide protein to make certain he can keep and bring together muscle. His favourite supply of protein is seafood, however he moreover consumes protein shakes, steak, turkey, hen, and eggs too. Ronaldo adjustments his breakfast food relying on the desires of training/video video games, however he has been stated to consume entire-grain cereal, egg whites, fruit juice, espresso, bloodless cuts, cheese, avocado toast, and fruit. For his first snack of the day, Ronaldo regularly enjoys fish and bread.

For lunch, Ronaldo likes fish or hen, entire-wheat pasta or a baked potato, and inexperienced vegetables. For his 2d snack of the day, he keeps it quick via consuming a protein shake to promote muscle recuperation after his vigorous education. For dinner, Ronaldo often enjoys his favored meal of Bacalhau à Brás. It is a Portuguese dish made from salted cod, onions, potatoes, scrambled eggs, black olives, and sparkling parsley. From time to time, Ronaldo moreover eats salads, rice, and beans. Again, he does now not devour those kinds of meals in a unmarried sitting, but he does devour tremendous substances like those to make sure that he performs nicely and recovers fast.

Now, even though that could be a nutrients ebook, do not be misled into believing that he eats now not whatever unstable because of the fact he's going to have a very good time birthdays with cake and on occasion has chocolate too. Therefore, if ninety five% of your food are healthful, a slice of cake will now not hold you back too much. However, have to you need to avoid eating junk food, you could have an advantage over individuals who do. Also, because of the fact one of the most important standards of this ebook is to make matters winnable, hold in mind having dark chocolate in preference to milk chocolate to make certain you have grow to be masses of antioxidants while you satisfy that chocolate yearning. Similarly, find natural cake mixture whilst baking a cake to know that the additives are better than the usual pre-made cake which has 50+ materials— hundreds of which may be tough to pronounce.

Lionel Messi's Weekly Eating Plan

Now, allow us to damage down Lionel Messi's meal plan, in keeping with Men's Health Magazine. A week earlier than a in shape, Messi decreases his carbohydrate consumption and will increase the amount of protein and water he consumes. Also, Lionel Messi eats vegetable soup with spices on the begin of food. Some spices Messi uses are chili powder, coriander, ginger, and turmeric. Without as many carbohydrates, Messi may also experience slightly a whole lot much less strength in the days leading as much as a endeavor. Cutting carbohydrates forces his frame to come to be greater green with the sugar ranges in his blood.

Once Messi reintroduces carbohydrates a day in advance than the sport and at the day of the sport, it'll increase his strength because of the carb loading. Messi's first-class dinner the day in advance than a activity carries meat (e.G., fish, chicken, or prawns), green greens, an orange, and potatoes. Six hours before healthy time, Messi eats porridge and egg whites. Then, ninety mins earlier than the game begins offevolved, Messi eats fruit. Now, do you want to visit this quantity thru beginning every week in advance than each undertaking to appearance consequences? Probably not. However, apprehend that the greater you are taking ingesting seriously, the extra it will help beautify your in-recreation overall performance.

So, do you be conscious any similarities among Ronaldo and Messi? They every consume healthy ingredients understanding that it will fuel their performances to ensure they will be the top notch. If you're questioning how pinnacle athletes like Cristiano Ronaldo teach within the gymnasium and at the pitch, make certain to grab the Understand Soccer collection ebook, Soccer Fitness. Here is a precis of Ronaldo's & Messi's meal plans need to you want to look lower back at them fast:

Cristiano Ronaldo

Sample Breakfast:

Whole-grain cereal, egg whites, and fruit

Sample Snack #1:

Tuna roll with lemon juice

Sample Lunch:

Chicken salad, inexperienced veggies, and a baked potato

Sample Snack #2:

Protein shake

Sample Dinner:

Turkey, beans, rice, and fruit

Lionel Messi

1 week in advance than a big in shape:

Meat (fish, fowl, or prawns)

Green greens

Vegetable soup with chili powder, coriander, ginger, and turmeric

The day before a big suit:

Meat (fish, chicken, or prawns)

Green veggies

Orange

Potatoes

Six hours in advance than healthful time:

Porridge

Egg whites

Chapter 14: What To Eat On Non-Training Playing Days

After studying about meals to consume in advance than and after training, let us talk what to consume on non-schooling days. A non-training day is an off day in which you do not have weightlifting, exercising, excessive conditioning for at least half of-hour, or a fit. On nowadays, you want a bargain much less strength from meals but although need to avoid being hungry and get higher genuinely.

Dairy (cheese, Greek yogurt, entire-fat milk, and cottage cheese) takes a long term to your frame to digest, so the superb times for a football participant to eat it are as part of your remaining meal of the day in the end interest or on off days in that you aren't education. Milk sugar, lactose, is a complex sugar this is difficult to digest and more time consuming than easy sugar for your body to breakdown. Also, because milk protein is 80% casein protein, that is the slowest digesting protein that takes up to 7 hours to digest, it's miles awesome to avoid dairy in advance than bodily sports activities. Remember, food is gasoline. Be positive to apply the quicker digesting meals earlier than and right now after video video games and hold the slower digesting food for while you skip long periods with out eating, the most apparent one being while you fall asleep.

You can have a look at greater approximately the macronutrients I intention to eat on off days, however I consume fewer carbs thinking about that I do no longer need as masses strength on off days. Furthermore, I eat extra fat to make sure I live whole, despite the truth that I actually have fed on plenty a great deal less food. Similarly, I typically tend to eat round 3,600 electricity in step with day on days I exercise and first-class three,000 energy on days I do no longer exercising to make sure my body has the electricity to perform once I am competing. So, what does this mean for you? Well, make sure to eat extra food on education days to beautify everyday overall performance and help healing but reduce the quantity you devour on off days to ensure you live at a amazing frame composition.

Additionally, the reason you need to consume extra fats is not first-class to stay complete, however to combat contamination. Inflammation takes region to your joints, ligaments, tendons, spine, and many others. Whenever hobby occurs. So, after days in which you exercised intensely, your frame may be stricken by contamination which creates physical pain and will increase the time your body should spend resting in location of getting organized for the game you want. As a quit end result, eating greater irritation stopping fat will make it a good deal less tough to come to be without a doubt recovered and get lower lower back on the sphere. According to Harvard Health Publishing, trans fats boom infection within the body, so we need to recognition on the unsaturated fat with anti inflammatory residences, in line with the American Journal of Clinical Nutrition. Consume fat like nuts, fish/fish oil, and olive oil to combat infection.

Nuts like almonds, walnuts, and pistachios are immoderate in protein, fats, and fiber and feature unsaturated fats, which assist lower your bad ldl cholesterol and lift your outstanding ldl cholesterol. Fish oil has omega-three fatty acids, which help hold your blood-fat ranges in an remarkable range, reduce stiffness, reduce the outcomes of bronchial bronchial asthma, growth focus, and decrease joint ache. Lastly, a have a study published inside the Journal of Nutritional Biochemistry found that the oleocanthal in olive oil had a huge effect no longer only on persistent contamination however furthermore on acute inflammatory strategies, much like the effects of nonsteroidal anti inflammatory pills (NSAIDs) like aspirin or ibuprofen (Motrin/Advil). Therefore, you can benefit the equal inflammation-reducing houses from olive oil because the unnatural, over the counter capsules, that have poor prolonged-time period aspect effects, particularly to your liver.

Furthermore, if you are someone who's constantly seeking out techniques to get an facet over your competition, stretching to your off days is a great way to preserve your muscular tissues flexible, have healthy joints, lessen your risk of damage, and beautify recuperation. Stretching permits inside the healing of muscle companies thru lengthening them and growing the amount of blood flow to them to get rid of the lactic acid. Lactic acid is created at the equal time as you use your muscles past the element they are used to jogging, which creates muscle pain the following day or . If studying extra about stretching pursuits you to beautify your restoration and dominate at the pitch, then take maintain of the Understand Soccer collection book, Soccer Fitness, to observe extra. Also, very mild exercising like walking will help to rid your frame of its soreness too.

In summary, the nice time to devour dairy is as a part of your final meal of the day assuming you're executed with all bodily hobby or are on an off day. Off days are a excellent time to reduce your carbohydrate consumption because of the fact you need lots much less electricity. Furthermore, ingesting extra fat on off days in the form of nuts, fish/fish oil, and olive oil will assist you live entire and decrease the quantity of inflammation to your body which lengthens the time it takes as a way to completely recover and get once more on the field. Lastly, a chunk of stretching and on foot will pass an extended manner to supporting to improve blood go along with the flow in your sore muscle mass a good way to lessen your restoration time extensively.

Chapter 15: Sports Drinks Vs. Water?

When: Ounces: Ounces-to-Bottles:

2-three Hours Before Activity   sixteen ounces.   About 1 Regular-Sized Bottle

15 Minutes Before Activity eight   oz. About half of Regular-Sized Bottle

During Activity   4 oz. Every 15-20 minutes About 2-three Large Gulps (1/four of a Regular-Sized Bottle)

After Activity   16-20 ounces   1 to at the least one-1/four Regular-Sized Bottles or 1 Large Bottle

So how plenty water ought to you drink? According to the National Collegiate Athletic Association (NCAA), right right here is the recommended amount of water to devour for a college athlete. Reduce the thing duration depending on your age:

Remember, how an lousy lot you need to devour is primarily based upon on the weather situations, and your stage of hobby on the field. Specifically, in case you are a goalkeeper gambling inside the cool climate of a overdue-fall activity, then eating a whole lot of water is not as crucial. The chillier temperature will restriction the amount you sweat, and goalkeepers are the least-active gamers at the arena. However, in case you are an outdoor midfielder who runs a ton, and you are playing in the heat summer time solar, then you definitely definitely definately need to double or triple the quantity of water you consume at halftime at some point of a game.

When you sweat and do bodily exercise, your body uses electrolytes. Although which could seem like a complex phrase, an electrolyte is a kind of salt. Sodium, potassium, chloride, calcium, magnesium, and phosphate are all common components of electrolytes. Electrolytes are vital for nerve and muscle characteristic; they participate in regulating bodily fluids, and they help manage blood strain. With this expertise, many businesses have created products geared toward supporting athletic basic normal performance. In precept, those liquids need to assist enhance your usual typical performance, but allow us to check what is definitely in a sports activities drink, and whether eating one on the identical time as gambling allows. Here is the label of a bottle of the precept sports drink logo:

The Good:

It has water and a few electrolytes (salt, sodium citrate, and monopotassium phosphate).

The Bad:

Sugar – It has a variety of sugar this is simplest beneficial if you are exercise strenuously for as a minimum 60 minutes or greater.

Dextrose – A faster-digesting form of sugar this is right now usable with the aid of your body. Again, except you are workout intensely for at least an hour, you do no longer want it.

Citric Acid – Adds flavor and acts as a preservative.

Artificial Flavors – Synthetic chemical substances that rate a wonderful deal tons less to deliver than finding natural belongings.

Modified Food Starch – Most usually derived from genetically modified corn, then altered to provide it a extra perfect texture.

Glycerol Ester of Rosin – a synthetic oil-soluble food additive called "E445" used to maintain oil in suspension in beverages.

Blue 1 – Linked to destructive chromosomes it is your genetic material. Each coloured sports activities sports drink has a one-of-a-type dye which negatively impacts your health.

Next, the British Medical Journal has published many articles revealing the reality about sports activities beverages. Specifically, drink whilst you are thirsty and do not waste your cash or energy on sports sports beverages—water is the higher choice as an alternative. The British Medical Journal team exposed that sports sports activities drink makers spent some of cash sponsoring much less-than-rigorous studies which advised thirst changed into not a high-quality guide to hydration and casting doubt on water because of the truth the beverage for staying hydrated. According to Fortune Business Insights, they assume the sports drink marketplace to attain $32.Sixty one thousand million thru 2026. Therefore, the identical businesses which may be telling us water is not appropriate sufficient are the equal agencies that income at the same time as we purchase their sports sports drinks.

In summary, water is the doctor recommended drink of choice for athletes. Avoid the overpriced sugar water with some precise sorts of salts which do now not advantage you a exceptional deal and function plenty of risky filler elements. Drink as you're thirsty to make certain you still be hydrated.

Chapter 16: General Nutrition Tips

This chapter is a capture-excited by way of matters that must be on this eBook but do no longer need a whole monetary disaster themselves.

1. Eat your meals so as.

2. Food on-the-cross.

3. Stay far from alcohol, smoking, pills, processed meals, and fast substances.

four. Use the remarkable salt.

five. Glass boxes > plastic bins.

First, maximum people are best worried with ingesting wholesome meals, however they do now not don't forget the order wherein they must eat the wholesome food. Say you have a healthy meal of natural bread, broccoli, hen, and a banana. Most humans eat the bread first due to the fact they have got now not eaten in a while, and their blood sugar is low. They consume most of the bread preceding to beginning on the alternative factors of their meal. They take bites of the whole thing; unfortunately, the broccoli is the final meals completed because of the reality they recognize it is healthy, however it their least preferred component on their plate. Eating within the order of carb, fruit, meat, vegetable is brilliant every proper in advance than a activity or right now after a game to growth your electricity levels for soccer or increase your blood-sugar levels after a exercise to make sure that you use greater of your meal to rebuild your muscle tissues.

However, ingesting in this order isn't always maximum inexperienced for the food which may be a long way from bodily exercising. If you are hours some distance from exercising or a football exercise/activity, then you definately have to opposite the order in that you devour your meals. You need to consume in order of vegetable, meat, fruit, grain. This guarantees that you will devour the slower-digesting food first. This will reduce the risk of a blood-sugar spike and make certain that you have a normal circulate of electricity for the subsequent severa hours, preceding to ingesting your subsequent meal. If you devour inside the contrary order, and you consume the quicker-digesting grains/carbs and fruit first, then your blood sugar will spike, extra of the meals can be saved as fats, your blood sugar will dip dramatically, and also you will become exhausted and function constrained electricity for the following few hours, till you devour all over again.

Explained greater scientifically, the higher the blood-sugar (i.E., glucose) degree on your frame, the greater insulin your pancreas releases to stability your blood-sugar stages. Insulin additionally breaks down fat and proteins for electricity. If your pancreas releases a whole lot of insulin, then it's far going to start breaking down all of your meals proper away, for this reason supplying you with some of power for an hour or so. This is fantastic if you may play soccer but bad if you will now not be energetic, due to the fact you can experience a large energy crash. Rapidly changing blood-sugar levels can purpose severe lengthy-term health troubles, like diabetes.

Second, make consuming wholesome winnable. By having meals to capture on-the-skip, you growth the possibilities you're making the right food alternatives. If you are a decide studying this ebook, consider grabbing the Understand Soccer collection e-book, Soccer Parenting, for proper now usable records to help your soccer participant carry out higher on the field and to beautify yourself notion helping them with football, even if you have by no means accomplished in advance than yourself. Here is a chart of healthful food prepared to eat or that take minimal education; You will be aware that most of the snacks are quit result and vegetables:

Third, there are various matters on the way to make it more difficult to be a fulfillment in football and existence. The sports activities activities so that it will prevent you from being the high-quality player you could be are ingesting, the usage of drugs recreationally, and smoking. These are want to-keep away from behavior as they may force you to spend time, cash, and intellectual power on things other than soccer and effect your health and staying energy on the world. Also, even though now not as glaringly lousy for you, processed meals and maximum rapid-food eating places will exceptional sluggish you down. Fries and a burger earlier than a recreation or containers of processed meals will handiest restriction your power, gradual your growth, lessen your performances, and decrease your frame's capability to get better. If you want to eat processed elements, aim to consume the herbal options. If you should grab fast-food, then stay with Chipotle or Pan era Bread.